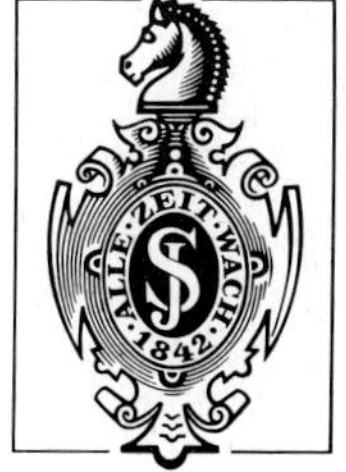

Varicocele and Male Infertility

Recent Advances in Diagnosis and Therapy

Edited by
E. W. Jecht and E. Zeitler

With the Collaboration of
W. Adam   H.-D. Adolphs   K. Amplatz   G. Antes   F. Barret
K.-H. Barth   J. M. Bigot   D. Brandl   W. Castaneda-Zuniga
F. Comhaire   K. H. Conrad   D. Djawari   A. Formanek   A. Gebauer
R. Grosse-Vorholt   S. G. Haider   A. T. Harahap   J. Haselberger
C. Helenon   R. Herzinger   B. Hilscher   W. Hilscher   N. Hofmann
O. P. Hornstein   R. Hubmann   R. Janson   E. W. Jecht   S. Kadir
H. Kasseckert   S. L. Kaufman   A. J. Keller   L. Knebel   P. M. Kövary
M. Kunnen   G. Ludwig   F. Lunglmayr   C. Meisel   R. Müller
H. Niermann   D. Passia   K. M. Pirke   E.-I. Richter   T. Riebel   P. Riedl
G. Schieferstein   C. Schirren   P. Schramm   K. M. Schrott   W. Seyferth
M. Simons   R. Sintermann   W. Stackl   G. Staehler   M. Thelen
M. Vandeweghe   A. Vermeulen   D. Völter   H. Vogel   H.-J. Vogt
L. V. Wagenknecht   L. Weißbach   R. I. White   H. Wokalek   J. Wutz
E. Zeitler   E. Zieglwalner   Ch. L. Zollikofer

Springer-Verlag
Berlin Heidelberg New York 1982

E. W. Jecht, Dr. med.
Dermatologische Universitäts-Klinik und -Poliklinik, Hartmannstr. 14, D-8520 Erlangen

E. Zeitler, Professor Dr. med.
Radiologisches Zentrum, Abteilung Diagnostik, Klinikum Nürnberg, Flurstr. 17, D-8500 Nürnberg

With 98 Figures

ISBN 3-540-10727-4 Springer-Verlag Berlin Heidelberg New York
ISBN 0-387-10727-4 Springer-Verlag New York Heidelberg Berlin

Library of Congress Cataloging in Publication Data. Main entry under title: Varicocele and male infertility. Includes bibliographical references and index. 1. Varicocele. 2. Varicocele—Surgery. 3. Infertility, Male. I. Jecht, E. W. 1939– II. Zeitler, E. (Eberhard), 1930– [DNLM: 1. Sterility, Male—Etiology. 2. Varicocele— Diagnosis. 3. Varicocele—Therapy. WJ 780 V299] RC898.V24   616.6   81-18324   ISBN 0-387-10727-4 (U.S.)   AACR2

Typesetting, printing and bookbinding: Konrad Triltsch, Würzburg
2127/3130-543210

Foreword

It is not surprising that so much investigation has been undertaken to establish the cause of childlessness, especially when the *potentia coeundi* of the male is not impaired. As long ago as 1957 the German Society for the Study of Fertility and Sterility was founded, embracing gynecology, andrology, and veterinary medicine. After its inception, meetings conducted in the spirit of its foundation were held every 2 years. This interdisciplinary, coordinated scientific work in the field of human reproduction achieved its value as a result of the stimuli provided by the permanent involvement of veterinary scientists.

After about 20 years of activity, the Society adopted a highly differentiated pattern of work-directions in the field of human and veterinary medicine. Since 1976 annual meetings have been held on the topic of animal and human reproduction. These meetings have proved of great value, especially in the area of comparative medicine, and have led to excellent interdisciplinary associations. One of the most evident successes was the first extracorporal fertilization in humans with subsequent embryo transfer and full-term pregnancy.

Gynecologists have found that in 40% of cases the cause of undesired childlessness rests with the male, and it is therefore no surprise that also in the field of andrology certain factors concerned with infertility have received great attention. Their exact scientific elaboration requires specific kinds of symposia. The Varicocele Symposium, held in Nürnberg on 15 and 16 March 1980 under the auspices and promotion of the German Society for the Study of Fertility and Sterility, was thus devoted to a single male disorder affecting fertility, a disorder that accounts for approximately 15% of male reproductive disturbances.

The present book, containing the proceedings of this symposium, deals with the multifarious aspects of treatment and diagnosis of the disorder. For the planning of the symposium, as well as for its organization and documentation, we have to congratulate Dr. E. Jecht. His excellent work deserves the gratitude of us all, and so it is not only in the name of the German Society for Study of Fertility and Sterility that these thanks are offered.

Kiel, November 1981 — Prof. Dr. Dr. h. c. K. Semm

Preface

The abnormal dilatation and tortuosity of the pampiniform plexus known as idiopathic varicocele is a condition rather common in men: according to the most recent investigations, its prevalence is 15% or more.

There is substantial evidence that varicocele impairs spermatogenesis and, consequently, semen quality, although contradictory data have been published recently. However, varicocele is considered to be the most frequent cause of male infertility.

All available data attest to the reversed blood flow in the internal spermatic vein(s) as being the factor actually detrimental to spermatogenesis in varicocele. However, reflux in the internal spermatic vein(s) has been demonstrated in patients suffering from reduced semen quality but without clinical evidence of varicocele. The presence of reversed blood flow in the internal spermatic vein(s) without varicocele (referred to as "subclinical varicocele") can only be detected employing methods such as Doppler sonography, thermography, and phlebography.

Doppler sonography is rapidly achieving the status of the screening technique for the detection of subclinical varicocele. Considered to be the method of first choice by some investigators, thermography requires time for the adaptation of the patient to room temperature and an experienced examiner. Systematic radiological examinations to detect and/or assess the extent of subclinical varicoceles have shown anomalies of the left internal spermatic vein in about 80% of the patients in whom a reflux was proven. Moreover, the phlebographic results demonstrate that a reversed blood flow is more frequently present in the right internal spermatic vein than previously suspected.

The treatment of varicocele had been exclusively surgical until the recent development of percutaneous transcatheter occlusion of the internal spermatic vein(s). This nonsurgical method represents a considerable achievement when compared to the requirements for surgical therapy such as general anesthesia and admittance to hospital. This monograph presents a comprehensive and concise description and evaluation of almost all techniques available for the detection and assessment as well as the treatment of (sub)clinical varicoceles. Particular emphasis is placed on the recent advances in Doppler sonography, thermography, phlebography, and percutaneous transcatheter occlusion of the internal spermatic vein. The complex relationship between varicocele and semen quality is thoroughly discussed. Data recently gathered in various centers showing the effect of nonsurgical treatment of varicocele on semen quality are presented in great detail.

It has been the editors' goal to provide the reader with an in-depth and well-planned volume covering "varicocele and male infertility". We believe that the presentation of the work of such a highly interdisciplinary gathering of noted investigators is an achievement in itself. It is our sincere hope that physicians involved in reproductive medicine, such as urologists, dermatologists, endocrinologists as well as radiologists and gynecologists, will find this first monograph on "varicocele and male infertility" instructive, helpful, and attractive.

Finally, it gives the editors great pleasure to thank Dr. WIECZOREK and his associates at Springer-Verlag for their advice and cooperation.

Erlangen, Nürnberg, October 1981   EKKEHARD W. JECHT
                                                    EBERHARD ZEITLER

Acknowledgments. The studies and the development of sclerotherapy were made with the assistance of the "Förderverein der Radiologie e.V., Nürnberg". The generous help of the following companies is gratefully acknowledged: Bayropharm GmbH, Köln; Glaxo Pharmazeutika GmbH, Bad Oldesloe; Hoechst Aktiengesellschaft, Frankfurt; Ichthyol-Gesellschaft Cordes, Hermanni & Co., Hamburg; Isotopen Dienst West GmbH, Dreieich bei Frankfurt; Organon GmbH, Oberschleißheim; Serono Pharm. Präparate GmbH, Freiburg.

Contents

VI. Results

VII. Discussion

List of Collaborators

W. Adam	Universitäts-Hautklinik Tübingen, Abt. Dermatologie II, D-8500 Nürnberg
H.-D. Adolphs	Urologische Klinik der Universität Bonn, D-5300 Bonn
K. Amplatz	Röntgendiagnostisches Zentralinstitut, Universitätsspital, CH-8091 Zürich
G. Antes	Radiologische Klinik und Poliklinik der Universität München, Klinikum Großhadern, Hartmannstraße 14, D-8520 Erlangen
F. Barret	Hôpital Tenon, Radiologic Department 4, rue de la Chine, F-75020 Paris
K.-H. Barth	John-Hopkins-Hospital, Department of Radiology, Baltimore, Maryland 21205, USA
J. M. Bigot	Hôpital Tenon, Radiologic Department 4, rue de la Chine, F-75020 Paris
D. Brandl	Dermatologische Universitätsklinik und Poliklinik Erlangen, Hartmannstraße 14, D-8500 Erlangen
W. Castaneda-Zuniga	Röntgendiagnostisches Zentralinstitut, Universitätsspital, CH-8091 Zürich
F. Comhaire	Department of International Medicine, Academisch Ziekenhuis, State University Gent, De Pintelaan 135, B-9000 Gent
K. H. Conrad	Dermatologische Universitätsklinik und Poliklinik Erlangen, Hartmannstraße 14, D-8520 Erlangen
D. Djawari	Dermatologische Universitätsklinik und Poliklinik Erlangen, Hartmannstr. 14, D-8520 Erlangen

A. FORMANEK	Röntgendiagnostisches Zentralinstitut, Universitätsspital, CH-8091 Zürich
A. GEBAUER	Radiologische Klinik und Poliklinik der Universität München im Klinikum Großhadern, Marchioninistr. 15, D-8000 München 70
R. GROSSE-VORHOLT	Radiologische Abteilung, Klinikum Nürnberg, Flurstraße 17, D-8500 Nürnberg
S. G. HAIDER	Anatomisches Institut der Universität Düsseldorf, Universitätsstr. 1, D-4000 Düsseldorf
A. T. HARAHAP	Universitäts-Hautklinik, Von-Esmarch-Str. 56, D-4400 Münster
J. HASELBERGER	Urologische Klinik, Klinikum Mannheim der Universität Heidelberg, D-6800 Mannheim
C. HELENON	Hôpital Tenon, Radiologic Department 4, rue de la Chine, F-75020 Paris
R. HERZINGER	Dermatologische Universitätsklinik und Poliklinik Erlangen, Hartmannstraße 14, D-8520 Erlangen
B. and W. HILSCHER	Institut für Hygiene der Universität Düsseldorf, Universitätsstr. 1, D-4000 Düsseldorf
N. HOFMANN	Andrologische Abteilung, Universitätshautklinik, Moorenstraße 5, D-4000 Düsseldorf
O. P. HORNSTEIN	Dermatologische Universitätsklinik, Hartmannstraße 14, D-8520 Erlangen
R. HUBMANN	Urologische Klinik der Universitätsklinik Hamburg, Martinistraße 52, D-2000 Hamburg
R. JANSON	Abteilung f. Radiologie und Urologie der Universität Bonn, D-5300 Bonn 1, Venusberg
E. W. JECHT	Dermatologische Universitäts-Klinik und Poliklinik Erlangen, Hartmannstr. 14, D-8520 Erlangen
S. KADIR	John-Hopkins-Hospital, Department of Radiology, Baltimore, Maryland 21205, USA
H. KASSECKERT	Universitäts-Hautklinik Tübingen, Abt. Dermatologie II, D-8500 Nürnberg
S. L. KAUFMAN	John-Hopkins-Hospital, Department of Radiology, Baltimore, Maryland 21205, USA

A. J. Keller	Krankenhaus St. Trudpert, Wolfbergallee 50, D-7530 Pforzheim
L. Knebel	Urologische Klinik, Klinikum Mannheim der Universität Heidelberg, D-6800 Mannheim
P. M. Kövary	Universitäts-Hautklinik, Von-Esmarch-Straße 56, D-4400 Münster
M. Kunnen	Department of Radiology, Academisch Ziekenhuis, State University Gent, De Pintelaan 135, B-9000 Gent
G. Ludwig	Urologische Klinik, Klinikum Mannheim der Universität Heidelberg, D-6800 Mannheim 1
G. Lunglmayr	Zentrales Institut für Radiodiagnostik, Allgemeines Krankenhaus d. Stadt Wien, Alsterstr. 4, A-1090 Wien
C. Meisel	Wiesenstraße 107, D-8500 Nürnberg
R. Müller	Dermatologische Universitätsklinik und Poliklinik Erlangen, Hartmannstr. 14, D-8520 Erlangen
H. Niermann	Universitäts-Hautklinik, Von-Esmarch-Straße 56, D-4400 Münster/Westfalen
D. Passia	Anatomisches Institut der Universität Düsseldorf, Universitätsstr. 1, D-4000 Düsseldorf
K. M. Pirke	Technische Universität München, Biedersteinerstraße 29, D-8000 München
E.-J. Richter	Radiologische Abteilung, Klinikum Nürnberg, Flurstraße 17, D-8500 Nürnberg
T. Riebel	Abteilung für Radiologie, Universitätskinderklinik Hamburg, D-2000 Hamburg
P. Riedl	Franz-Josefs-Kai 3, A-1010 Wien
G. Schieferstein	Universitäts-Hautklinik Tübingen, Abteilung Dermatologie II, D-7400 Tübingen
C. Schirren	Abteilung für Andrologie, Hautklinik der Universität, Martinistraße 52, D-2000 Hamburg 20
P. Schramm	Hautklinik der Johannes-Gutenberg-Universität Mainz, D-6500 Mainz

K. M. SCHROTT	Urologische Klinik, Maximiliansplatz, D-8520 Erlangen
W. SEYFERTH	Radiologische Abteilung Klinikum Nürnberg, Flurstraße 17, D-8500 Nürnberg
M. SIMONS	Department of International Medicine, Academisch Ziekenhuis, State University Gent, De Pintelaan 135, B-9000 Gent
R. SINTERMANN	Technische Universität München, Biedersteiner-straße 29, D-8000 München 40
W. STACKL	Zentrales Institut für Radiodiagnostik, Allg. Krankenhaus der Stadt Wien, Alsterstr. 4, A-1090 Wien
G. STAEHLER	Radiologische Klinik und Poliklinik der Universität München im Klinikum Großhadern, Marchioninistr. 15, D-8000 München
M. THELEN	Abteilung für Radiologie der Universität Mainz, D-6500 Mainz
M. VANDEWEGHE	Department of International Medicine, Academisch Ziekenhuis, State University Gent, De Pintelaan 135, B-9000 Gent
A. VERMEULEN	Department of International Medicine, Academisch Ziekenhuis, State University Gent, De Pintelaan 135, B-9000 Gent
D. VÖLTER	Urologische Abteilung, Krankenhaus St. Trudpert, Wolfbergallee 50, D-7530 Pforzheim
H. VOGEL	Urologische Klinik der Universitätsklinik Hamburg, Martinistraße 52, D-2000 Hamburg
H.-J. VOGT	Technische Universität München, Biedersteiner-straße 29, D-8000 München 40
L. V. WAGENKNECHT	Urologische Klinik der Universitätsklinik Hamburg, Martinistraße 52, D-2000 Hamburg 20
L. WEISSBACH	Urologische Klinik der Universität Bonn, D-5300 Bonn
R. I. WHITE, Jr.	John-Hopkins-Hospital, Department of Radiology, Baltimore, Maryland 21205, USA
H. WOKALEK	Universitäts-Hautklinik, Hauptstraße 7, D-7800 Freiburg

J. WUTZ   Spitzwegstraße 22, D-8520 Erlangen

E. ZEITLER   Radiologisches Zentrum, Abt. Diagnostik, Klinikum Nürnberg, Universität Erlangen-Nürnberg, Flurstraße 17, D-8500 Nürnberg

E. ZIEGLWALNER   Dermatologische Universitätsklinik und Poliklinik Erlangen, Hartmannstraße 14, D-8520 Erlangen

CH. L. ZOLLIKOFER   Röntgendiagnostisches Zentralinstitut, Universitätsspital, CH-8091 Zürich

I. Epidemiology

Epidemiology of Idiopathic Varicocele

J. WUTZ

Idiopathic varicocele is defined as the dilatation and prolongation of the veins of the pampiniform plexus. Idiopathic varicoceles are predominantly located on the left side: The percentages reported by various investigators differ between 70% and 100% for the left-sided varicocele, between 0% and 23% for varicoceles on both sides, and between 0% and 9% for the right-sided varicocele [7].

It is well known that patients with a varicocele represent a relatively large group among men consulting an infertility service. Meyhöfer and Wolf reported a prevalence of 10% [9], Hornstein of 38% [6], and Amelar and Dubin of 39% [1]. A large range of percentages has been reported by various investigators for the prevalence of idiopathic varicoceles in the normal population [2, 8, 10, 11].

In 1976, I checked 3490 men of military age for a varicocele during physical examinations for military service. For this investigation, the presence of a varicocele was accepted only if a soft scrotal varicosity of dilated veins was palpable. Elongation of the left or the right hemiscrotum and/or elongation and thickening of the funiculus spermaticus without palpable scrotal varicosity were not included as varicocele.

There were 181 young men with a varicocele among the 3490 men examined, corresponding to 5.1% [12]. All varicoceles were located on the left side. None of the 181 men had previously known about the varicocele. Four men reported irregular and diffuse subjective symptoms in the genital and/or inguinal area.

When comparing my results with the data accumulated over the years in the military service, a striking difference was found: Among 3 906 948 men of military age, there were 75 877 men with a varicocele, corresponding to 1.942%. A wide range of percentages was evident when the total number of 3 906 948 was broken down according to the examining physicans: The minimal prevalence was found to be 0.527%; the maximal, 6.197% [3]. It is very unlikely that this large difference is due to real differences between the prevalence of varicocele in different populations. It is my assumption that the varying prevalence of varicocele among military men is caused by the varying degree of thoroughness among different physicicans, which is common knowledge with respect to the genital area.

The prevalence of varicoceles found by other investigators supports the assumption that the prevalence seen in the German military service is too low, due to insufficient physical examination [2]. Bailey and Love reported a prevalence of 5–10% in men 15–35 years old; Johnson et al. [8] found a prevalence of 10% (number and age not indicated), while Øster found a prevalence of 16.2% among 837 students age 10–19 years [10]; Steeno et al. described a prevalence of 14.7% in 4067 students 12–35 years old [11]. I examined 184 students (age 15–16 years) and found 21 of them to have a varicocele, corresponding to a prevalence of 11.4%.

The prevalence of varicoceles appears to be ––within limits ––age dependent. According to most investigators, varicoceles are rarely seen before puberty. Demel reported that 60% of varicoceles develop between the ages of 15 and 25 years [4]. According to Ebner, 2% of varicoceles develop before the age of 14, 52% between the ages of 15 and 25, 33% between the ages of 26 and 35, and 13% after the age of 35 years [5]. Øster found the following distribution of varicocele: age 10 years and less, 0%; age 10 years, 5.7%; age 14 years, 19.3% [10]. The corresponding figures of Steeno are as follows: 12 years, 5.0%; 15 years, 15% [11]. In conclusion, there seems to be a greater prevalence of varicoceles in recent years. This increase is most likely due to a greater awareness of the consequences for semen quality attributed to varicoceles and a more thorough examination of the scrotal organs, particularly by experienced investigators.

References

1. Amelar RD, Dubin L (1973) Male infertility, current diagnosis and treatment. Urology 1:1
2. Bailey H, Love D (1973) A short practice of surgery. Lewis, London
3. Beiträge zur Wehrmedizinalstatistik. Institut für Wehrmedizinalstatistik und Berichtswesen, Hefte 19, 24, 30
4. Demel R (1926) Chirurgie des Hodens und des Samenstranges. Neue Dtsche Chir 36:422
5. Ebner E (1929) Zur Klinik und Therapie der idiopathischen Varicocele. Dtsch Z Chir 219:148
6. Hornstein OP (1973) Kreislaufstörungen im Hoden-Nebenhodensystem und ihre Bedeutung für die männliche Fertilität. Andrologie 5:119
7. Jecht E (1977) Varikozele und Fertilität. Zbl Haut Geschlechtskr 138:177
8. Johnson DE, Pohl DR, Rivera-Correra H (1970) Varicocele. An innocuous condition? South Med J 63:34
9. Meyhöfer W, Wolf J (1960) Varikozele und Fertilität. Dermatol Wochenschr 142:1116
10. Øster J (1971) Varicocele in children and adolescents. Scand J Urol Nephrol 5:27
11. Steeno O, Knops J, Declerck L, Adimoelja A, Van De Voorde H (1971) Prevention of fertility disorders by detection and treatment of varicocele at school and college age. Andrologia 8:47
12. Wutz J (1977) Über die Häufigkeit von Varikozelen und Hodendystopien bei 19jährigen Männern. Klinikarzt 6:319

II. Basic Aspects

Pathogenesis of Varicocele

G. Ludwig

The logically inaccurate designation *varicocele*, defined by Ambroise Paré in the sixteenth century as a "vascular plexus filled with melancholic blood", is taken to mean a phlebectasia of individual or all regions of the pampiniform plexus. To understand the pathogenesis of this phlebectasia, one must consider a large number of etiological factors responsible individually or in combination for the genesis of a varicocele.

Knowledge of normal anatomy and physiology is the prerequisite for understanding the etiology and pathogenesis of the disease.

Anatomy

The venous drainage of the testis takes place chiefly via a deep network of veins and a superficial network of veins anastomosing with it. The deep venous network consists of the external spermatic vein, the deferens vein, and the internal spermatic vein. The pampiniform plexus is formed from the testicular vein, the epididymal vein, and the accompanying veins. It drains near the inguinal ring after these veins have joined to form the internal spermatic vein, which opens almost perpendicularly on the left side into the left renal vein. The right internal spermatic vein joins the vena cava at an angle of 30–40° about 4 cm below the junction point of the right renal vein. The extended pampiniform plexus constitutes the anatomical substrate of varicocele.

In the literature, numerous factors have been accorded responsibility for the pathogenesis of idiopathic varicocele. Nevertheless, many points remain under dispute. All authors agree on a clear preponderance of varicocele on the left side. Ivanissevich [12] found idiopathic variocele on the left in 4470 cases. Oster [26] also found an exclusive localization on the left in his 837 cases. Various other authors report a strong preponderance of occurrence oh the left, but also found bilateral varicoceles and varicoceles on the right only in an average of 2% – 3% of the cases [9, 16, 20, 29, 32]. However, it must be borne in mind that according to Åhlberg et al. [1] the right spermatic vein opens into the right renal vein in 10% and even more frequently according to Brown et al. [2]. Comparable junctional conditions to those on the left side would then be present. Grillo-Lopez [8] made the interesting discovery in 1971 that a situs inversus was present in three cases of isolated varicocele on the right side.

It could be concluded from all these investigations that an idiopathic varicocele very seldom occurs only on the right side, if at all, under normal drainage conditions into the vena cava.

The possible etiological explanations for the almost exclusive occurrence of idiopathic varicocele on the left side are listed below:

a) Congenital and hereditary weakness of the connective tissue and of the vessel walls [9, 10, 15], which predisposes to status varicosus.
b) Defective development of the cremaster muscle and congenital atonia of the scrotum [7].
c) Raised hydrostatic pressure due to greater length of the left internal spermatic vein [9, 30].
d) Unfavorable inflow conditions at the junction with the left renal vein due to: 90° junction [23, 25], raised pressure of the renal vein compared to the vena cava [19, 28], or additional elevation in pressure by clamping of the renal vein at the angle between the aorta and the superior mesenteric artery [10, 15, 24].
e) Compression from outside by lymph nodes [25], or a course between inferior mesenteric artery and aorta [5, 18]
f) Congenital absence of valves or closure insufficiency of valves present [1, 3, 11, 13, 14, 21, 28, 31].

Point f) requires elucidation. The congenital absence or closure insufficiency of valves was postulated as the cause for the development of a varicocele as early as 1909 [11], but this hypothesis was rejected in the 1930s, in some cases on the basis of inexact investigation [25]. However, this etiological factor gained increasing attention in recent years as a result of investigations of pathological anatomy on autopsy material and the introduction of transfemoral retrograde phlebography [3, 14, 21].

The nature and position of the valves or their absence or insufficiency were demonstrated very inhomogeneously, and in some cases in a contradictory fashion. Mellin [22] reported in 1970 that the internal spermatic vein has no valves at all; this had already been established by the Göttingen anatomist Henle in the middle of the nineteenth century. Ivanissevich and Gregorini [13] assumed valvular insufficiencies were an etiological factor in the genesis of varicocele in 1918 although they were unable to prove the presence of valves. Gösfay [6], Åhlberg [1], Brown [2], and Kohler [17] were also merely able to confirm radiologically the lack of valves in the left internal spermatic vein by retrograde and anterograde phlebography. Comhaire and Kunnen pointed out in 1974 that a junctional valve can sometimes be lacking in men [3].

In 1974 we investigated the drainage conditions of both internal spermatic veins to clarify the position of valves in the two internal spermatic veins. We also hoped to be able to give at least a hypothetical explanation from the anatomical conditions found for the almost exclusive occurrence of an idiopathic varicocele on the left [21]. The average length of the spermatic vein was 42 cm. Two or more spermatic veins were almost always found. They frequently anastomosed with each other in a manner resembling a rope ladder (Fig. 1). Six of the 50 autopsied cadavers had had an untreated varicocele on the left side. This was shown by the markedly phlebectatic pampiniform plexus and could be confirmed by retrospective anamnestic studies. A

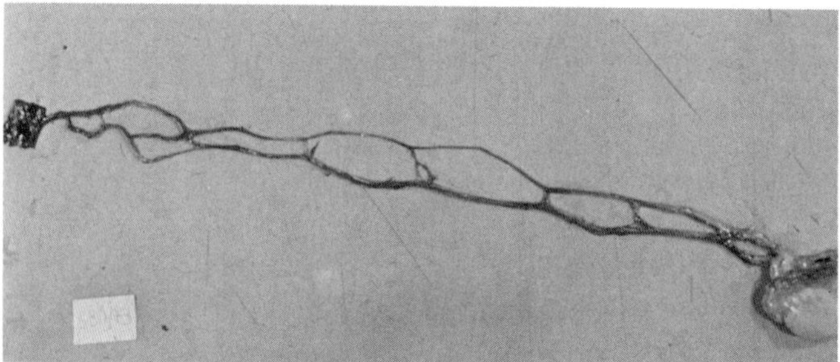

Fig. 1. Left testis with dissected internal spermatic veins and their ropeladder-like anastomoses up to the junction with left renal vein

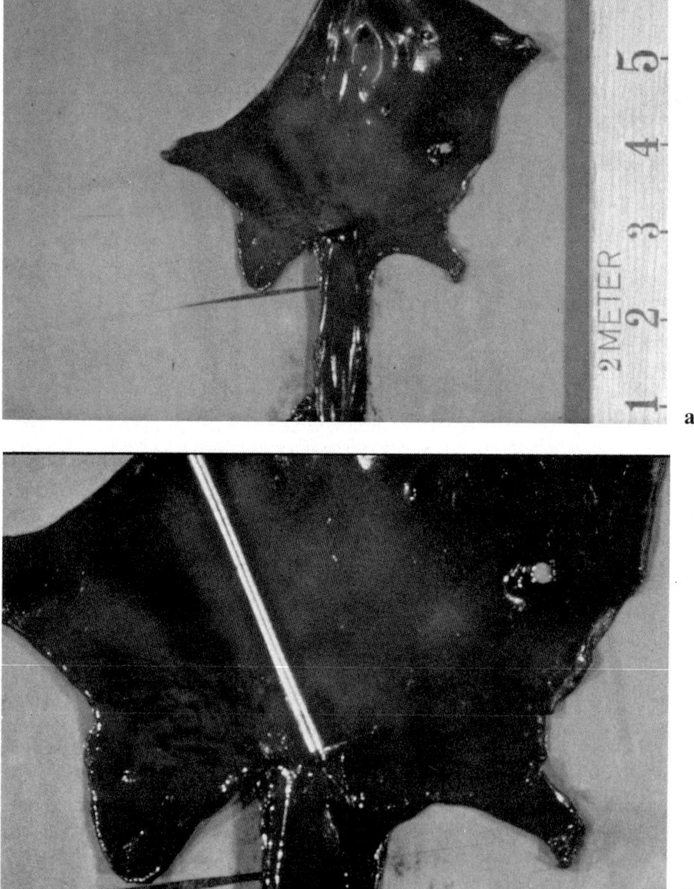

Fig. 2. a Site of opening of the left internal spermatic vein into the renal vein (both vessels are cut open). The junctional valve is to be clearly recognized. The suprarenal vein joins opposite (above). **b** The junctional valve of the left internal spermatic vein is raised by a probe

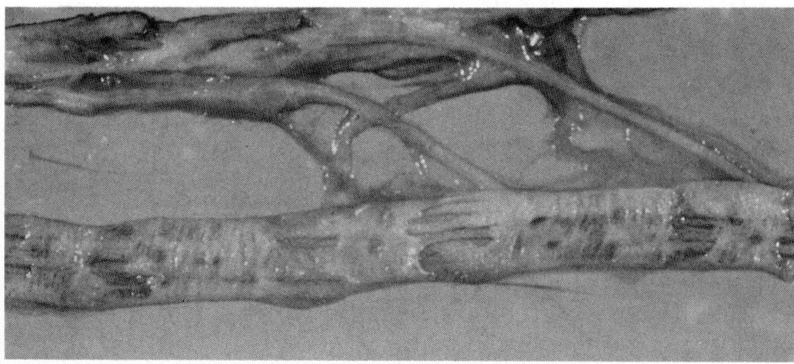

Fig. 3. Several valve pairs of the left internal spermatic vein in the suprainguinal region

valve at the junction with the renal vein was found in all 50 cases (Fig. 2). In 18 cases the suprarenal, vein opened into the renal vein exactly opposite the opening of the the spermatic vein. All six cases in which varicocele was present belonged to this group; the junctional valve documented in Fig. 2 was the only valve in these six cases. In 38 additional cases, a further three to eight valve pairs were found in the left internal spermatic vein. These were located chiefly in the groin region and higher (Fig. 3).

A junctional valve alone was present in a total of 12 cases, and, as stated above, a varicocele was found in six of these cases. In the right spermatic vein, which was on average 4.5 cm shorter than the left spermatic vein and opened into the inferior vena cava at an average angle of 40°, four to ten valve pairs were found in all cases. A junctional valve was always present even here.

In order to study a larger number of veins in patients with a varicocele, we not only ligated the internal spermatic vein according to Bernardi in 20 patients but also excised a 10–12 cm long section reaching from the internal inguinal ring upwards (thus corresponding to the region in which the most valves were otherwise found). We did not find a valve in any of these 20 cases (as in the six cadaver varicoceles).

Table 1. Valves of the spermatic vein (own results)

Material:		50 autopsy preparations: of these, six varicocele patients. 20 internal spermatic vein sections excised in an operation according to Bernardi
Results:	Left:	All 50 had a junctional valve at the renal vein
		The junctional valve was the only valve in 12 cases
		All six varicocele patients had only this junctional valve
		A further three to eight valve pairs were found in the suprainguinal region in 38 cases
		The suprarenal vein opened exactly opposite the junction point of the internal spermatic vein in 18 cases
		20 excised portions of the internal spermatic veins of living varicocele patients had no valves in the suprainguinal region where most valves are otherwise situated
	Right:	Both the junctional valve and several valve pairs in the suprainguinal region in all 50 cases

Our results, summarized in Table 1, show that the left spermatic vein always has a junctional valve, but that this is occasionally the only venous valve. The right spermatic vein always has several valves.

The suprarenal vein frequently opens opposite the junction with the spermatic vein. This leads to turbulences in the blood flow which can promote a junctional valve insufficiency, which *then* induces development of a varicocele on the left when no additional valves in the inguinal region catch the backflow of blood. This can explain why idiopathic varicocele of the testis is almost always found on the left side. Under normal drainage conditions into the vena cava, a large number of valves would always have to be insufficient to develop a varicocele on the right side.

In the presence of an isolated varicocele on the *right* side, the following possibilities would accordingly have to be excluded: (1) a symptomatic cause such as a renal tumor or another tumor which has grown forward into the retroperitoneum, (2) an abnormal opening of the right internal spermatic vein into the right renal vein, and (3) a situs inversus.

A bilateral varicocele is based either on an additional symptomatic cause on the right side or an abnormal opening of the right spermatic vein into the right renal vein or, as assumed by Haensch and Hornstein [9] as well as Ludvik [20], suprapubic anastomoses between the left and right pampiniform plexus. However, these would likewise have to be without valves or with valvular insufficiency.

The insufficiency of the junctional valves leads to a reflux of blood from the left renal vein into the left spermatic vein and to congestion and a phlebectasia of the pampiniform plexus. If this condition persists for a long time, anatomical fixation of the phlebectasia occurs by hypoplasia of the elastic fibers and hypertrophy of the media musculature of the vein walls analogous to formation of leg varices. Szypura and Meyer [29] as well as Dathe et al. [4] were able to demonstrate corresponding changes in histological preparations.

According to the investigations by Shafik et al. [27], there occurs in addition an atrophy of the "fasciomuscular pump," a physiological unit consisting of the cremasteric fascia and the external and internal spermatic fasciae which surround the spermatic cord and actively promote venous reflux. If this pump ceases to function, the veins of the spermatic cord and of the pampiniform plexus can stretch without impediment by relaxation in the presence of venous reflux from the internal spermatic vein with valvular insufficiency.

Summary

Idiopathic varicocele of the testis, which occurs almost exclusively on the left, may possibly be based etiologically on an insufficiency of the junctional valve at the junction with the renal vein. This can be promoted by turbulences in blood flow by the suprarenal vein which opens exactly opposite. If further valve pairs are absent in the remaining course of the spermatic vein, as appears to be the case in varicocele patients, there is a reflux of blood from the renal vein back to the pampiniform plexus with a phlebectasia of the venous plexus. If this phlebectasia persists for a long time, there is an anatomical fixation by hypoplasia of the elastic fibers and hypertrophy of the media musculature of the vein walls as in formation of leg varices.

A congenital and hereditary weakness of the connective tissue and the vessel walls doubtless play a role in determining the degree of predisposition. The raised hydrostatic pressure due the great length of the perpendicularly rising vessel can also have a promoting effect.

Due to the pressure of the phlebectatic vein wall, there is in addition an atrophy of the fasciomuscular pump, which otherwise actively promotes venous reflux. The typical signs of idiopathic varicocele then result. Impairment of fertility may ensue by way of mechanisms which have not yet been precisely and definitively clarified.

References

1. Åhlberg NE, Bartley O, Chidekel N, Fritjofsson A (1966) Phlebography in varicocele scroti. Acta Radiol [Diagn] (Stockh) 4:517
2. Brown JS, Dubin L, Becker M, Hotchkiss RS (1967) Venography in the subfertile man with varicocele. J Urol 98:388
3. Comhaire F, Kunnen M (1976) Selective retrograde venography of the internal spermatic vein: A conclusive approach to the diagnosis of varicocele. Andrologia 8:11
4. Dathe G, Heine H, Nickel C (1976) Pathomorphose der Plexusvenen bei Varikozele. Med Welt 27:1564
5. El Sadr AR, Mina E (1950) Anatomical and surgical aspects in the operative management of varicocele. Urol Cutaneous Rev 54:257
6. Gösfay S (1959) Untersuchungen der Vena spermatica interna durch retrograde Phlebographie bei Kranken mit Varikozele. Z Urol 52:105
7. Goljanitzky JA (1926) Zur Frage der Entstehung und chirurgischen Behandlung der Venenerweiterung des Samenstrangs. Arch Klin Chir 141:481
8. Grillo-Lopez AJ (1971) Primary right varicocele. J Urol 105:540
9. Haensch R, Hornstein O (1968) Varikozele und Fertilitätsstörung. Dermatologia 136:335
10. Hornstein O (1964) Zur Klinik und Histopathologie des männlichen Hypogonadismus. III. Mitteilung: Hodenparenchymschäden durch Varikozelen. Arch Klin Exp Dermatol 218:347
11. Istomin E (1914) Zur Frage der operativen Behandlung der Varikozele. Zentralbl Chir 41:93
12. Ivanissevich O (1960) Left varicocele due to reflux. J Int Coll Surg 34: 742
13. Ivanissevich O, Gregorini H (1918) Uno nuovo operacio para anar el varicocele. Sem Med 25:575
14. Janson R, Weissbach L (1978) Zur Phlebographie der Vena testicularis bei Varikozelen-Persistenz bzw. Rezidiv. ROEFO 129:485
15. Klika, M (1955) Die neuen Ansichten über die Ätiologie und Therapie der idiopathischen Varikozele. Urol Int 2:142
16. Klosterhalfen H, Schirren C, Wagenknecht LV (1979) Pathogenese und Therapie der Varikozele. Urologe [A]18:187
17. Kohler FP (1967) On the etiology of varicocele. J Urol 97:741
18. Leger L, Proux C, Duranteau M (1957) Phlébographie rénale et cave inférieure par injection intraparenchymateuse. Press Med 67:141
19. Lopatkin NA (1973) Pathogenic foundation of new method of operative treatment of varicocele (in Russian, English abstr). Urol Nefrol (Mosk) 38:31
20. Ludvik W (1970) Varikozele und Fertilität. Act Urol 1:184
21. Ludwig G, Jentzsch R, Peters HJ, Fiene R (1975) Die Klappen der Vena spermatica interna. (Ein Beitrag zur Pathogenese der idiopathischen Varikozele). Act Urol 6:89
22. Mellin P (1971) Diskussionsbemerkung. Verhandlungsbericht der deutschen Gesellschaft für Urologie (Baden-Baden 1970). Springer, Berlin Heidelberg New York, p 262
23. Meyhöfer W, Wolf J (1960) Varikozele und Fertilität. Dermatol Wochenschr 41:1116
24. Moldovan J (1974) Varicocel "idiopatic" prin reflux hidrostatic san varicocel "boala" prin baray mecanic aortomezenteric (in Rumanian, English abstr). Chirurgia (Bucharest) 23:257

25. Oberndorfer S (1931) In: Henke-Lubarsch: Handb. spez. Path., vol VII, part 3. Springer, Heidelberg Göttingen, p 743
26. Oster J (1971) Varicocele in children and adolescents. Scand J Urol Nephrol 5:27
27. Shafik A, Khalil AM, Saleh M (1972) The fasciomuscular tube of the spermatic cord. Br J Urol 44:147
28. Smirnoff OL (1929) Varicocele sinistra idiopathica. Z Urol 23:850
29. Szypura E, Meyer J (1971) Structure of the walls of the normal testicular vein and in varicocele (in Polish, English abstr). Folia Morphol (Warsz) 30:223
30. Völter D (1972) Die idiopathische Varikozele aus andrologischer Sicht. Fortschr Med 90:683
31. Völter D, Wurster J, Aeikens B, Schubert GE (1975) Untersuchungen zur Struktur und Funktion der Vena spermatica interna – Ein Beitrag zur Ätiologie der Varikozele. Andrologia 7:127
32. Weissbach L (1978) Die idiopathische Varikozele. – Eine Übersicht. Extracta Urol 1:255

The Varicocele: Clinical Aspects

H. WOKALEK

Introduction

Even though the varicocele was first described as early as 1541 by Ambroise Paré [7], reports on research into its clinical aspects are totally missing for almost 400 years. This is probably because, until recently, no connection was made between the varicocele and its functional affect upon male fertility. Only since Tulloch's report in 1952, on successful varicocele surgery resulting in restored fertility, and his assumption of pathogenetic interaction between advanced varicocele and inhibited fertility [9], do we recognize the varicocele as one etiologic factor for oligo- or asthenospermia and the often resulting infertility.

While there is evidence of improved spermiogram parameters up to normal fertility after surgery, connections between the presence of a varicocele and male infertility are not of such certainty that total restoration of normal fertility may be insured after surgery.

Since limited fertility is not necessarily caused by a varicocele, the degree of fertility cannot be gauged exclusively by the clinical degree of a varicocele.

With the frequent connection between the presence of a varicocele and infertility it has become extremely important to recognize the often very discrete clinical symptoms of the varicocele and to render clinically a first diagnostic orientation of its degree.

The varicocele is often discovered when a patient with a varicocele consults an andrologist about his infertility. The patient is seldom aware of the varicocele, its relationship to infertility, and the possibility of cure, so that he lacks all motivation for an operation when told of the necessity for surgery.

Nomenclature and Definition

We define a varicocele as a varicosity of the pampiniform plexus. The constitutional (idiopathic or primary) varicocele is to be differentiated from the symptomatic one.

The constitutional varicocele usually occurs at the end of puberty, or shortly thereafter [8], in the left part of the scrotum (Fig. 1). This predominance, as well as its hemodynamic and anatomic varieties, is discussed later in this volume.

The symptomatic varicocele may be a leading symptom for a neoplastic process within the small pelvis and also for the possible presence of tumors within the limits of venous drainage of the testes, usually at the intra- and retroperitoneal regions of the kidneys.

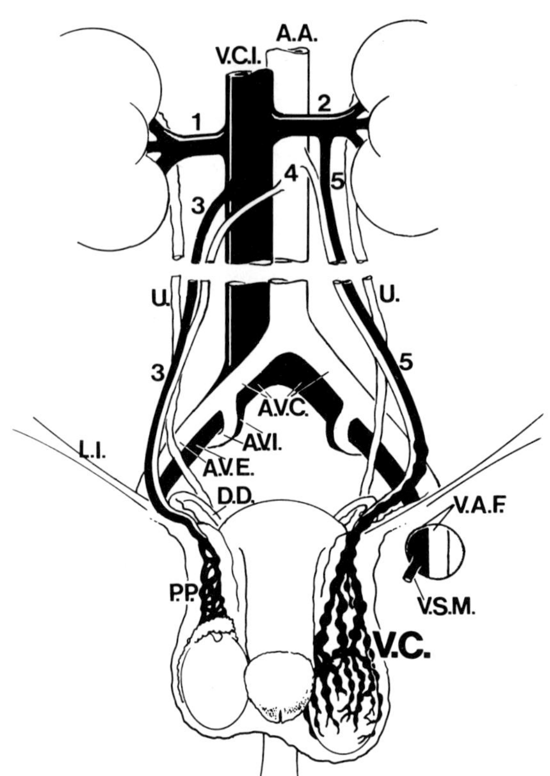

Fig. 1. The schematic drawing shows the venous drainage of the testes. A.A., aorta abdominalis; V.C.I., vena cava inferior; A.V.E., arteria and vena iliaca externa; A.V.C., arteria and vena iliaca communis; A.V.I., arteria and vena iliaca interna; V.A.F., vena and arteria femoralis; V.S.M., vena saphena magna; V.C., varicocele; U., ureter; L.I., ligamentum inguinale; P.P., plexus pampiniformis; D.D., ductus deferens; 1, vena renalis dextra; 2, vena renalis sinistra; 3, vena testicularis (spermatica) interna dextra; 4, arteriae testiculares dextra et sinistra; 5, vena testicularis (spermatica) interna sinistra.

Since the mode of origin of the symptomatic varicocele is not related to regular anatomic conditions, there will be no preference for either testis. The symptomatic varicocele appears in both testes with equal frequency, normally developing quite rapidly, without favoring certain age groups.

This means, one first has to consider the presence of a symptomatic varicocele with its suppressing process in the tight drainage region of a varicose dilated testicular vein; whether the patient has reached old age or has not yet reached puberty.

We rarely see clinically manifest varicose dilations at the pampiniform plexus in boys before puberty. The apex of varicocele manifestation with regard to clinical symptoms and effect lies in the third decade, with the exception of the age-independent symptomatic varicoceles.

Clinical Relevancy of the Varicocele

The varicocele is seldom very painful. When standing the patient will simply notice an increased congestion in the region of the upper scrotum, as well as a small degree of pulling. Often a patient will complain of a heaviness in the scrotum, but very rarely about pain in the inguinal region.

A varicocele may occasionally lead to psychological disturbances, especially if the varicocele is of such a size that the genital region appears deformed and abnormal.

Some authors also see connections between advanced stages of the varicocele and complaints in the urogenital region in the sense of a vegetative urogenital syndrome analogous to the generation of varicoceles in the female region of the ligamenta uteri and its consequent "pelvis congestion" complaint.

Clinically manifest varicoceles are usually associated with a weak venal vessel system and are often accompanied by varicosis of the lower extremities and hemorrhoids [3].

Clinical Diagnosis

Clinical diagnosis of the varicocele is based on observation and palpation with the patient standing astride or in a supine position. Many varicoceles can be diagnosed simply by observation (Fig. 2). During palpation of the astride standing patient the congestion in the pampiniform plexus will increase with intraabdominal pressure (Valsalva test). If a varicocele is present a definite venous convolution of the pampiniform plexus can be palpated in the upper part of the scrotum.

In extreme cases the entire scrotal sac will have the feel of "a bag of worms". Light pressure may release overfilled veins. The idiopathic varicocele usually presents no constricting impediment in draining. In extreme cases the normally crinkled scrotal skin will be stretched flat and will appear thin. The testis in the varicose side, when palpated, will feel smaller and softer in comparison to the other one, and descends lower.

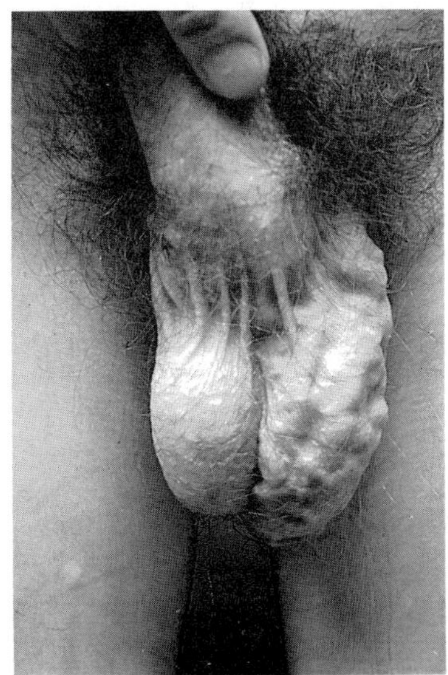

Fig. 2. Clinical aspect of an idiopathic varicocele.

The congested veins empty in the supine patient to such extent that the condition cannot always be diagnosed. But as soon as the patient stands the palpating hand of the physician will feel quite definitely the retrograde return of the venous blood into the meshed plexus.

The clinical diagnosis of a varicocele by palpation must be complemented by a spermatological examination to define the extent of the dysfunction. Spermacytologic as well as sperma-biochemic examinations should be performed.

It is to be assumed that there is a correlation between (a) the risk of damage of spermiogenesis and the accompanying risk of diminishing fertility and (b) the duration of a varicose condition. In extreme cases increasing testical atrophy can be expected [2].

Divisional Systems for Grading the Varicocele

Clinically, the degree of venal insufficiency cannot be determined with total accuracy. The best method to determine the extent of the insufficiency is phlebography.

To date, a reliable method has not been developed to correlate the degrees of varicosity and the effect on male fertility, nor are we able to define comparable diagnostic results, which would be useful with respect to follow-up.

Table 1

Class I:	large varicocele; the affected testis is considerably lower than on the contralateral side; and the patient complains of symptoms such as pain, dragging sensation and noticeable testicular atrophy;
Class II:	small, asymptomatic varicoceles; the testis usually does not hang any lower than normal; and the man often has not noticed its presence; and
Class III:	varicocele is intermediate in size between the other two classes and symptomatic [5].

Table 2

Grade I:	a "grape-sized mass" above the testis, which refills after compression;
Grade II:	the mass of the varicocele equals the size of the testis; and
Grade III:	the venous mass fills the hemiscrotum, usually extending up to the anulus inguinalis superficialis; the testis is displaced toward the septum scroti; and the varicocele is detectable by visual inspection alone [10].

Table 3

Grade I:	palpable scrotal varicosity of less than 1 cm in diameter and with reflux during a Valsalva maneuver;
Grade II:	pronounced varicocele mass with a diameter of 1–2 cm; and
Grade III:	the venous mass fills the hemiscrotum, is easily visible at a distance, and has a diameter greater than 2 cm at the time of positive pressure reflux [1].

Table 4

Varicocele A:	palpable, but not visible, prolongation, dilation and/or convolutions of the veins around the testis;
Varicocele B:	palpable and visible varicosity; and
Varicocele C:	pronounced changes, making differentiation of the testis difficult, and/or the presence of subjective symptoms [6].

In Tables 1–4 several suggestions for a grading method are collected from the literature. These grading systems are subjective and may suffice for a rough orientation on clinical divisions but are inadequate for an objective analysis aiming for a longitudinal or cross-cut profile. The safest method for establishing the extent of venal insufficiency is phlebography, the technique of which is in the foreground of this symposium.

Differential Diagnosis

One must differentiate between the idiopathic varicocele and the following conditions:

1. A hydrocele testis, which differs from the varicocele by its taut elastic consistency and positive diaphaneity.
2. Varix nodes below the inguinal ligament, which may imitate a varicocele condition upon palpation. In such cases, sounds can occasionally be evidenced with auscultation.
3. A scrotal hemangioma, which has a spongy consistency. In contrast to cases of varicocele, the Valsalva manoeuvre will be negative.
4. Lipomas along the vas deferens, which can be differentiated from the varicocele simply by palpation. Lipomas have a firm consistency and cannot be evacuated by pressure.
5. A scrotal hernia, which has a dough-like consistency. Palpation often reveals no connection with the ductus deferens.

Factors concerning differential diagnosis between idiopathic and symptomatic varicocele are provided by (a) localization and (b) time of manifestation and the length of time needed to develop the full clinical manifestation of the disease.

The localization on the right side with rapid development, especially in advancing ages, should arouse suspicion of a tumor. In such cases further diagnostic procedures including X-ray investigation are indicated.

References

1. Dubin L, Amelar RD (1970) Varioceles size and results of varicocelectomy in selected subfertile man with varicocele. Fertil Steril 21:606–609
2. Heite H-J, Wokalek H, Pfrieme B (1980) Männerheilkunde: Andrologie. Gustav Fischer. Stuttgart, pp 230–234

3. Hornstein OP (1973) Kreislaufstörungen im Hoden- und Nebenhodensystem und ihre Bedeutung für die männliche Fertilität. Andrologia 5:119–125
4. Ivanissevich O (1960) Left varicocele due to reflux. Experience with 4470 operative cases
   in forty-two years. J Int Coll Surg 34:742–755
5. Lewis EL (1950) The Ivanissevich operation. J Urol 63:165–167
6. Øster J (1971) Varicocele in children and adolescents. Scand J Urol Nephrol 5:27–32
7. Paré Ambroise (1541) Les œvres d'Ambroise Paré, Dixième Edition: 323
8. Steeno O (1972) Varicocele en Infertiliteit. Tijdschr Geneeskd 28:1313–1315
9. Tulloch WS (1952) A consideration of sterility factors in the light of subsequent pregnancies. II. Subfertility in the male. Trans Edinburgh Obstet Soc 194:29–34
10. Uehling DT (1968) Fertility in men with varicocele. Int J Fertil 13:58–60

Orchipathia e varicocele

O. P. HORNSTEIN

Valvular insufficiency of the left internal spermatic vein resulting in dilatation of the pampiniform plexus is the most common cause of varicocele. Some of the mechanisms entailing subsequent damage of the testicular tissue will be discussed here. Doubtlessly, the key to a better understanding of the complex pathogenesis of testicular injury lies in the special gonadal system.

The unique vascular supply of the testicles is the consequence of the descensus testium during fetal life, whereby the internal spermatic artery, as the longest organ artery of the body, represents, so to speak, the Ariadne thread of the descended gonad. The intrascrotal position of the testicles is a precondition of physiological hypothermia ensuring both normal proliferation and maturation of spermatozoa in the seminiferous tubules and the epididymal duct, respectively. The abdominoscrotal difference of body temperature in the male amounts to 2.0–2.5 °C; in some mammals to even more [6, 10, 11, 12, 31]. For maintenance of the intrascrotal hypothermia, the specialized vasculature of the funiculus spermaticus as well as the anatomical structure of the scrotum with tunica dartos is essential. The scrotum and spermatic cord act as a combined thermoregulatory unit which is disturbed after the occurrence of varicocele.

Brief Anatomical Remarks

To understand the varicocele-borne damage to testicular and epididymal structures we must look briefly at the principles of vascular supply of the male gonadal system. Each testicle is furnished by three arteries, the internal spermatic artery, the artery of ductus deferens, and, by taking into account some anastomotic bridges, the cremasteric artery (sive external spermatic artery). Venous reflux from the gonads is subject to a similar anatomical tripartition whereby the bulk of veins, after leaving the testicles, form a pampiniform plexus (i.e., like the tendrils of a vine), which closely surrounds the screw-shaped distal portion of the internal spermatic artery. The pampiniform plexus mainly collects the blood for both the internal spermatic vein and the deferential vein; the cremasteric vein(s) lead to the proximal femoral vein. This dividing is like a functional "watershed" of venous reflux since the blood of the pampiniform plexus, traversing a long intraabdominal distance, reaches the renal vein, whereas the blood collected by the cremasteric veins, after only a short distance, runs extraabdominally into the femoral vein. Some anatomical variability of the divided gonadal venous system may be the main reason for varying clinical findings in idiopathic varicoceles, so that some varicocele remains functionally compensated, i.e., the spermatogenesis is not significantly impaired.

In the 1950s, Harrison established the hypothesis [10, 12] that the very close anatomical interrelationship between the helical portion of the internal testicular artery and the sponge-shaped pampiniform plexus may make possible some heat exchange like a physical "reflux cooling system". A transfer of caloric energy from the warmer arterial to the cooler venous blood coming from the hypothermic testicles means the arterial blood will flow into the gonads in a precooled condition. This thermoregulatory "counterstream principle" has been verified experimentally in animals [6, 10, 11, 12, 31], whereas in the human no direct measurements of the funicular blood temperature have been performed as yet. Of course, such a thermoregulatory mechanism can only operate if the rewarmed venous blood returns to the heart with proper speed, otherwise the arteriovenous temperature gradient cannot be maintained. In the varicocele, however, the rewarmed blood flows so slowly that the intervascular caloric gradient may dissolve and the arterial blood may pour into the testicle without "precooling".

Moreover, the helical shape of the internal testicular artery is assumed to have, as shown in the ram [30], some significance for slowing down the speed as well as lowering the pressure of blood in the distal artery before entering the testicle. Whether or not some of the pulsating energy will be transmitted to the vascular wall of the surrounding plexus, as supposed by Barnett et al. [1] particulary in marsupials, has not yet been examined in the human. In any case, the upright position of man predisposes him ontogenetically to develop disorders of the peripheral venous system, including varicocele. In other words, "homo erectus" is in particular dependent on functional mechanisms which enable him to compensate the "physiologic orthostase" in the testicular veins. According to Shafik [27] the cremasteric muscle fibers constricting the spermatic cord normally are prone to support the hemodynamics of venous reflux.

Obviously, man is subject to a multitude of constitutional factors that may favour a state of orthostatic dysregulation of circulation in the low pressure blood system. From this view and in addition to the well-known asymmetry of the testicular venous system, the high prevalence rate of varicocele-bearing males in the population will be explicable.

Histology of Varicocele-Borne Testicular Damage

The altered blood circulation in the pampiniform plexus has some consequences for the testicular as well as epididymal functions. From some spermatological findings, in particular abnormalities of the tail and midpiece development, can be deduced [22, 23] that maturation of spermatozoa in the epididymal duct deteriorates at first. Later on, the spermiogenetic epithelium in the testicles is also involved so that in advanced stages of testicular damage a rather typical finding can be observed in testicular biopsies. The histology may offer such a characteristic picture that even without knowledge of clinical or spermatological data the diagnosis of an *orchipathia e varicele* can be made with some certainty [13].

Table 1. Histological findings of testicular biopsies in males with varicocele

Tubular:	Predominant but noncharacteristic lesions (nearly every stage of tubular insufficiency)
Interstitial:	Oedema and sclerosis (by increased reticulin and collagen fibers) of interstitium. Sclerosing involution of Leydig cells. Occasionally focal hyperplasia of uninvolved Leydig cells associated with clusters of degenerated Leydig cells.
Vascular:	"Hyaline adventitia sclerosis" (nonspecific) of small vessels (arterioles, capillaries). Dilatation and hyperemia of venules. Thickness and sclerosis of venous vessel walls. Structural changes of arteriovenous anastomoses.

The most typical criteria of the varicocele-borne orchipathy are *not* the degenerative and regressive lesions of the seminiferous tubules, although they appear predominant in the biopsy specimens. Of more significance for recognizing the varicocele-borne testicular destruction are minor changes in the interstitial tissue as well as some deformities of the venules surrounding the tubules and underlying the tunica albuginea, the area from which biopsy specimens usually are taken. In 13 out of 16 males with left-sided varicocele biopsy specimens of both testicles showed the parenchyma was damaged to a very similar extent [13].

Most *tubules* show an increased desquamation and disarrangement of spermatocytes and spermatids which progressively diminish. In advanced stages of testicular damage some tubules may loose even the spermatogonia and harbor only some residual Sertoli cells. Multinuclear giant cells (as a rule derived from spermatids) can often be found. In parallel to the increasing depopulation of the spermiogenetic epithelium a marked hyaline fibrosis of the tubular walls with shrinkage

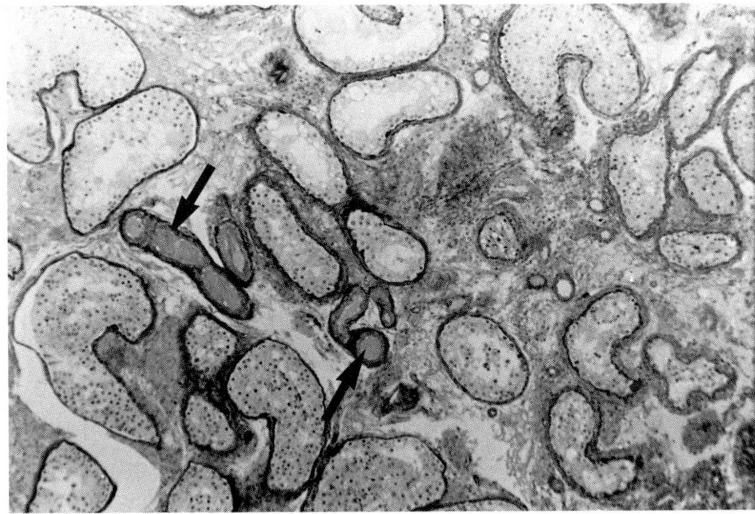

Fig. 1. Testicular biopsy. Interstitial edema, dilatation of small veins (↑). Separated tubules with diminution of seminiferous epithelium. van Gieson, × 45

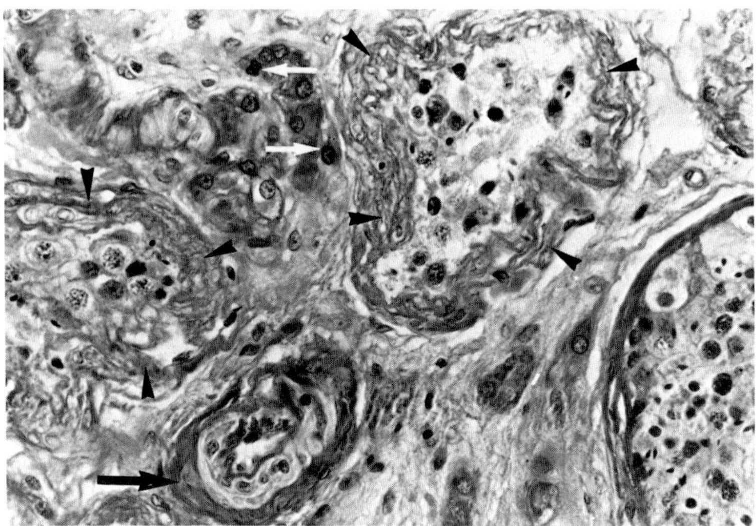

Fig. 2. Testicular biopsy. Peritubular fibrosis (▲) with advanced involution of spermatids and spermatocytes. Hyaline fibrosis surrounding a small shunt vessel (↑). van Gieson, × 45

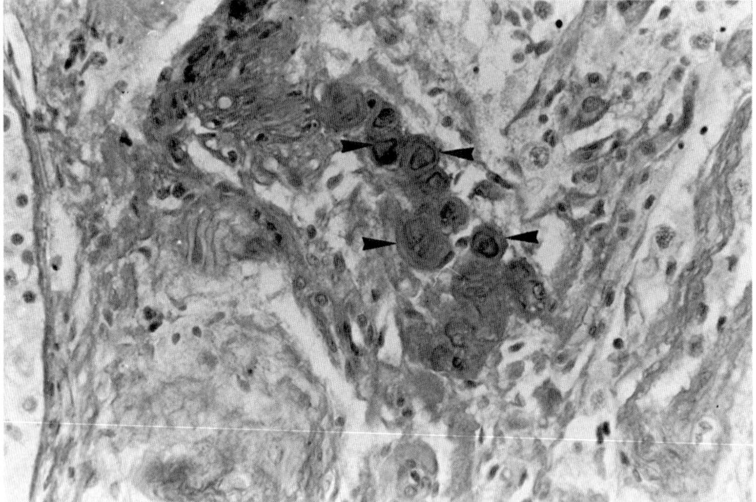

Fig. 3. Testicular biopsy. Pericellular sclerosis of Leydig cells with nuclear degeneration (▲). Minor fibrosis of the adjacent interstitial tissue. van Gieson, × 280

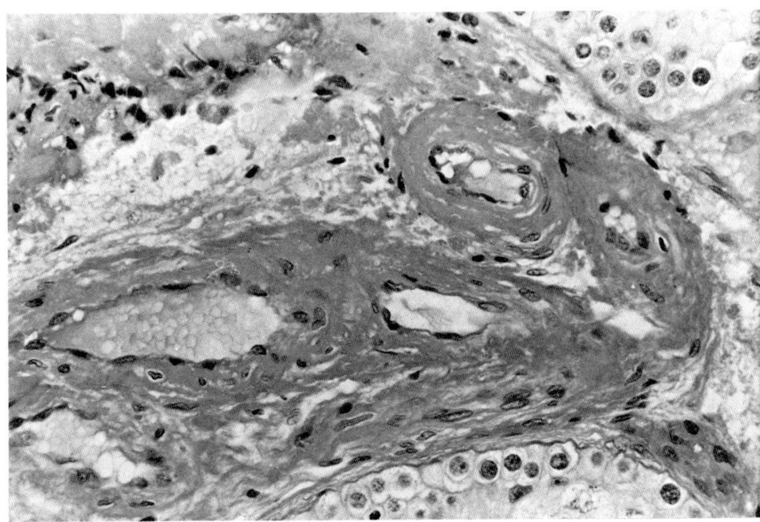

Fig. 4. Testicular biopsy. Cluster of venules with hyaline fibrosis of the vessel walls. Between seminiferous tubule (upper margin) and vessels there are some degenerated Leydig cells embedded in collagenous fibres. van Gieson, × 280

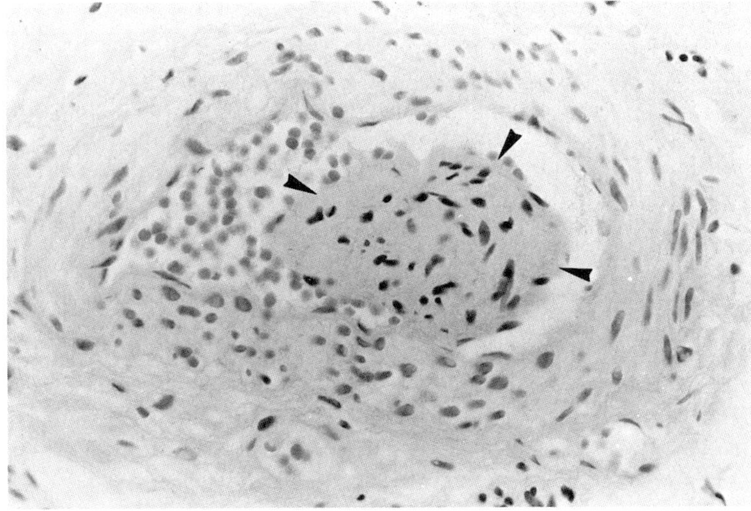

Fig. 5. Testicular biopsy. Small vein partially occluded by fibrous residuals of organized thrombus (▲). H & E, × 280

of the lumina occurs. It should be mentioned, however, that this type of tubular fibrosis can also be seen in testicular damage of very different origin. Obviously, the peritubular sclerosis entails a severe impairment of the intratubular metabolism and transmural transport system of hormonal and metabolic supply to and from spermiogenetic cells.

In the *interstitium* an edema with dilated and markedly hyperaemic venules usually will be found. The clustered Leydig cells are separated by the edema and a dense pattern of reticulin and collagen fibers as well, which wall in the single Leydig cells. This embedding causes progressive involution of the majority of Leydig cells which may fuse with adjacent peritubular fibrosis. Interestingly, some Leydig cells (in particular at the border of degenerated cell clusters) do not show any abnormalities and may even aggregate to islets like a hyperplasia. This focal increase of Leydig cells could be found in more than a third of our testicular biopsies with varicocele-induced sclerosis of the remaining interstitial cells. In my opinion the hyperplasia is the morphological expression of an hormonal attempt to compensate the destruction of Leydig cells by elevated gonadotrophic stimulation.

Vascular damage with marked thickening and sclerosis of small veins can mainly be found adjacent the tunica albuginea, representing a direct sign of venous hypostasis in the testicular parenchyma. Phlebosclerosis also covers the adventitia layers where hyaline cuff-shaped fibrosis surrounding the vessels may take place. Occasionally, some arteriovenous glomus vessels show considerable perivascular fibrosis and proliferation of the fibromyogenous inner wall with narrowing of the luminal space.

It should be mentioned that arteriovenous shunt vessels functioning as a by-pass for tissue microcirculation [3, 28] can also be found in testicles without varicocele. In varicocele-borne orchipathia, the peculiar remodel of glomus vessel structure appears to be of some significance. The alteration of glomus vessels probably is due to some decompensation of their bypass function as a consequence of an elevated back-pressure in the blood collecting veins.

Concluding Remarks

From the histological findings can be deduced that the varicocele-borne orchipathia begins in the interstitial tissue as a consequence of chronic venous hyperaemia with long-standing edema and increasing fibrillar sclerosis of many Leydig cells resulting in cellular obstruction. In a similar way fibrosis of the tubular walls inducing progressive involution of the intratubular spermatic cells occurs.

In our opinion, *three main pathomechanisms* are involved in the pathogenesis of the so-called orchipathia e varicocele [13]:

1. An increasing dystrophy of the testicular parenchyma caused by interstitial as well as peritubular fibrosclerosis.
2. A severe hypoxydose in the spermatic tubules and interstitial tissue due to an impeded exchange of oxygen and CO_2.
3. Long-standing blood hyperthermia which may indirectly injure the metabolism of the spermiogenetic epithelium.

Nevertheless there is some histological evidence that the Leydig cells remain more resistent against the elevated intratesticular temperature, since some normally appearing or even focally aggregated Leydig cells, probably induced by gonadotrophic hyperstimulation, can be found.

Whether or not the pool of Leydig cells originating in an abnormal tissue environment will have normal endocrine function is a question not yet exactly answered. Interestingly, in varicocele-bearing males decreased levels of plasma testosterone [4, 19, 26] as well as an increase of the LH excretion in urine [20] have been observed. Jecht et al. [17] were able to demonstrate an altered response of plasma testosterone levels to GnRH stimulation. Furthermore, in the seminal fluid of varicocele patients lowered contents of acid prostate phosphatase [25] and fructose [21] have been reported.

Finally, it should be mentioned that even some months after a varicocele operation the levels of testosterone in the peripheral venous blood have been shown to drop markedly from the preoperative state [16]. It may be possible that some Leydig cells remain in the preoperative state of insufficiency even after the elimination of the abnormal back-pressure of the venous blood.

References

1. Barnett CH, Harrison RG, Tomlinson JDW (1958) Variations in the venous systems of mammals. Biol Rev 33:442–487
2. Bohnstedt RM (1961) Fertilitätsstörungen bei Varikozelen und nach Hodendystopien und Leistenbruchoperationen. Z Geburtshilfe 157:156–161
3. Clara M (1956) Die arterio-venösen Anastomosen, 2nd edn. Springer, Vienna
4. Comhaire F, Vermeulen A (1975) Plasma testosterone in patients with varicocele and sexual inadequacy. J Clin Endocrinol 40:824–829
5. Curri SB, Tischendorf F, Maggi GC (1956) Experimentelle Untersuchungen zur Histophysiologie und -pathologie der arterio-venösen Anastomosen (nach Lebendbeobachtungen am Kaninchenohr). II. Mitt. Der Einfluß venöser Stauung, kreislaufwirksamer Pharmaka und der Vagotonie auf das Mikrooszillogramm. Acta Neuroveg 14:149–159
6. Dahl EV, Herrick J. F. (1959) A vascular mechanism for maintaining testicular temperature by counter-current exchange. Surg Gynecol Obstet 108:697
7. Glezerman M, Rakowszczyk M, Lunenfeld B, Beer R, Goldman B (1976) Varicocele in oligospermic patients: Pathophysiology and results after ligation and division of the internal spermatic vein. J Urol 115:562
8. Haensch R, Hornstein O (1968) Varicocele und Fertilitätsstörung. Dermatologica 136:335–349
9. Hanley HG, Harrison RG (1962) The nature and surgical treatment of varicocele. Brit. J Surg 50:64–67
10. Harrison RG (1952) Functional importance of the vascularization of the testis and epididymis for the maintenance of normal spermatogenesis. Fertil Steril 3:366–375
11. Harrison RG (1966) Male infertility. The anatomy of varicocele. Proc R Soc Med 59:763–765
12. Harrison RG, Weiner JS (1948) Abdomino-testicular temperature gradients. J Physiol (Lond) 107:48 P–49 P
13. Hornstein O (1964) Zur Klinik und Histopathologie des männlichen primären Hypogonadismus. III. Mitt. Hodenparenchymschäden durch Varicocelen. Arch Klin Exp Dermatol 218:347–383
14. Hornstein OP (1973) Kreislaufstörungen im Hoden-Nebenhodensystem und ihre Bedeutung für die männliche Fertilität. Andrologia 5:119–125
15. Jecht E (1978) Varikozele und Fertilität. Zentralbl Haut Geschlechtskrankh 138:177–187

16. Jecht E, Brandl D. Varicocele Operation and Endocrine Parameters (see page 106)
17. Jecht E, Glatz W, Becker H, Hornstein OP (1977) Hormonale Aspekte der Impotentia coeundi. Hautarzt [Suppl] 28:303–304
18. Johnson DE, Pohl DR, Rivera H (1970) Varicocele: An innocuous condition? South Med J 63:34–36
19. Marberger M, Frick J (1973) Zur Ätiologie der Spermiogeneseschädigung bei der Varikozele: Untersuchungen über den Plasmatesteronspiegel in der Vena spermatica. Urol Int 28:377–384
20. Mauss J, Börsch G (1974) Immunochemical assay of follicle-stimulating and luteinizing hormones in the unconcentrated urine of sub- or infertile males. Acta Endocrinol (Copenh) 74:631
21. Mauss J, Schach H, Scheidt J (1974) Andrologische Untersuchungen bei subfertilen Männern vor und nach Varicocelenoperation. Hautarzt 25:394–398
22. MacLeod J (1965) Seminal cytology in the presence of varicocele. Fertil Steril 16:735–757
23. MacLeod J (1969) Further observations on the role of varicocele in human male infertility. Fertil Steril 20:545–563
24. Meyhöfer W, Wolf J (1960) Varikozele und Fertilität. Dermatol Wochenschr 142:1116–1121
25. Raboch J, Żahor Z, Homolka J. Varicocele and the function of testes. Zit. nach 13
26. Raboch J, Stárka L (1971) Hormonal testicular activity in men with a varicocele. Fertil Steril 22:152–155
27. Shafik A (1973) The cremasteric muscle. Role in varicocelogenesis and in thermoregulatory function of the testicle. Invest Urol 11:92–97
28. Staubesand J (1959) Funktionelle Morphologie der Arterien, Venen und arterio-venösen Anastomosen. In: Ratschow A. Angiologie: Thieme, Stuttgart, pp 23–82
29. Steeno O, Knops J, Declerck L, Adimoelja A, Van de Voorde H (1976) Prevention of fertility disorders by detection and treatment of varicocele at school and college age. Andrologia 8:47–53
30. Waites GMH, Moule GR (1960) Blood pressure in the internal spermatic artery of the ram. J Reprod Fertil 1:223–229
31. Waites GMH, Moule GR (1961) Relation of vascular heat exchange to temperature regulation in the testis of the ram. J Reprod Fertil 2:213–224
32. Wutz J (1977) Über die Häufigkeit von Varikozelen und Hodendystopien bei 19jährigen Männern. Klinikarzt 6:319–320

Histological, Morphometrical, and Enzyme Histochemical Studies on Varicocele Orchiopathy

N. Hofmann, B. Hilscher, D. Passia, W. Hilscher, and S. G. Haider

Introductory Remarks on Clinical Aspects

In cases of varicocele, the clinical diagnosis is based on the nature of the scrotal varicosis and its associated characteristics, which may be as important in diagnosing this disease as the peculiar findings of the veins themselves. These characteristics are scrotal asthenia and low and horizontal position of the affected testicle, which is diminished in size and altered in consistency depending on the duration and degree of the vascular disturbance. Inguinal hernias, hemorrhoids, varicosis of the legs, and the overall leptosomatic constitution of the patients are further indications.

The varicocele is classified according to the scheme of Steeno et al. [10]. This scheme has been further developed in our clinic to differentiate between the plexus type and the testicular vein type of varicocele. The reflux, clinically determined by the Valsalva test, is also confirmed by the results of the Doppler examination. Transfemoral venous catheterization is performed in clinically doubtful cases.

Usually the spermatological findings and the results of hormonal analyses are in agreement with the clinical diagnosis. However, there are some exceptions; for example, the true varicocele cases, in which peritesticularly localized well-spread venous anastomoses may exist, providing a sufficient outstream of the testicular venous blood in spite of the reflux of the plexal veins. On the other hand, varicoceles may combine with other testicular disorders, of which chronic noninfectious orchitis [5] is a major problem of the intended operation. In this respect the kallikrein test (N. Hofmann and G. Ebert, Kallikrein in der diagnostischen Abklärung von Spermatogeneseschäden, unpublished work), prior to the operation, has proved to be a useful clinical test.

For the reasons above, testicular biopsies are performed rarely in cases of varicocele, providing a rather limited number of sections for morphological studies. Our studies were performed histologically, morphometrically, and enzyme histochemically, employing normal and semithin sections. With the help of these combined techniques new morphological aspects were studied.

Histological and Morphometrical Studies on Spermatogenesis

In typical cases of varicocele, spermatogenesis is attacked in the adluminal compartment of the seminiferous tubules, whereas the basal compartment remains normal for a certain time; the length of time cannot be predicted on the basis of pres-

Table 1. Number of germ cells and Sertoli cells in 50 cross sections of seminiferous tubules from two cases of varicocele and one normal testis [7]

	Cells/100 μm circumference	Varicocele				Normal testis
		II.°		III.°		
		right	left	right	left	
Spermatogonia	A_{dark}	0.15	0.21	0.02	0.03	0.39
	A_{pale}	2.69	2.12	1.33	1.32	2.00
	A_{long}	0	0	0	0	0.01
	B	0.26	0.43	0.03	0.03	0.59
Spermato-cytes	Pl.-cyg.	1.15	1.44	0	0.05	1.89
	Pachyt.	4.48	5.01	0	0	5.50
Spermatids	Round	3.13	3.79	0	0	5.09
	Elongated	2.52	2.68	0	0	3.46
Sertoli cells		2.31	2.07	6.85	5.91	2.63

ent knowledge. The determining factor leading to the impairment of basal spermatogenesis seems to be the damage of the arterial and arteriolar vessels of the testicles in the course of the venous disease. This will be discussed later.

The results of histological and morphometrical studies on spermatogenesis in cases of varicocele are as follows (see Table 1):

1. The counts of the A-dark spermatogonia are reduced to some extent [7]. However, this reduction is not so severe as in other serious disorders of spermatogenesis [3, 4]. The slight reduction is found on both sides, even in cases of sole left-sided varicocele.
2. At an early stage the counts of the spermatogonia of the A-pale type may be increased. This can be seen from sections of the right testicle, which clinically

Table 2. Mean area, circumference, and diameter of the walls of cross sections of seminiferous tubules [1]

Seminiferous tubules		Epididymal occlusion	Varicocele		Normal testis
			II.°	III.°	
		$n = 20$	$n = 20$	$n = 20$	$n = 50$
Area (μm_2)	$\overline{m}$	22 377.8	24 255.1	9 538.0	21 402.8
	s	7 597.8	9 235.7	2 991.7	7 335.4
Circumference (μm)	$\overline{m}$	59.9	646.0	377.0	521.4
	s	98.7	96.3	67.4	78.2
Diameter of tubular walls (μm)	$\overline{m}$	6.66	7.18	15.3	4.82
	s	1.9	1.9	2.4	1.4

showed a low-graded reflux, while on the left side a varicocele II° was found showing a conspicuous renotesticular reflux. This phenomenon of compensatory increase of spermatogenesis can be observed in cases showing high spermatozoa counts in spite of extended varicoceles. The spermatogonia of the A-pale type survive, even in cases of long-standing and serious varicoceles. However, according to our clinical results it is rather doubtful that spermatogenesis can be restored after operation in these cases.

3. Nuclear dysplasias of the spermatogonia, i.e., giant nuclei, multinucleosis, and degenerative lesions, were rarely found.
4. The reduction of I-spermatocytes is linked with reduced numbers of A-dark spermatogonia.
5. The characteristic finding is the reversible break of spermatogenesis/spermiogenesis at the stage of round and/or elongated spermatids [9]. This break is caused by exfoliation of single cells or cell plugs with dislocated nuclei of Sertoli cells. According to these different patterns of exfoliation, immature cells may be found in semen in varying accounts. Thus it can be postulated that varicocele orchiopathy begins with a disturbance of Sertoli cell function.
6. The degree of thickening and hyalinization of the boundary tissue of the seminiferous tubules (Table 2) is correlated to the stage of the disorder of spermatogenesis/spermiogenesis, as shown in our morphometrical results.

Enzyme histochemical Studies

Intratesticular varicosities could be demonstrated employing enzyme histochemical reaction for adenosine triphosphatase (ATPase), as shown in Fig. 1. The intensity of

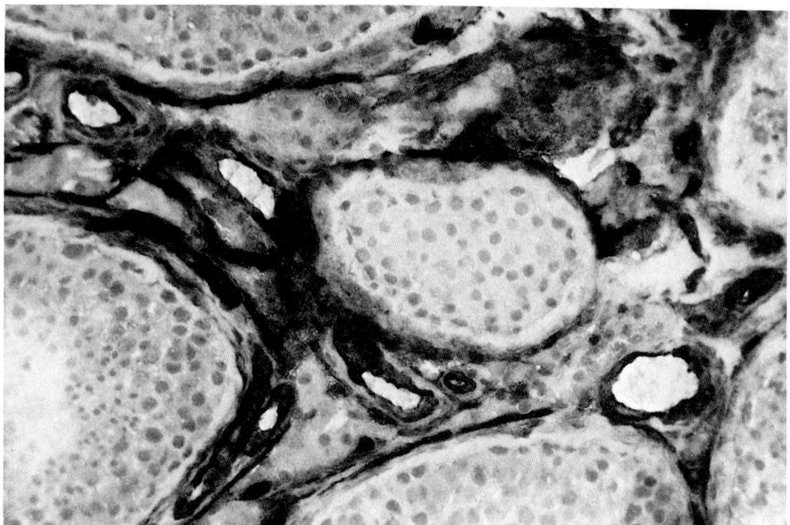

Fig. 1. Intratesticular varicosis in a case of varicocele shown by ATPase reaction

ATPase activity was reduced in some areas of the boundary tissue of the seminiferous tubules. In the same sections LDH activity also decreased to a varying degree [8].

The enzymatic activity of thiamine pyrophosphatase (TPPase) is a "marker" of the Golgi apparatus and the connected endoplasmic reticulum [8]. In the Sertoli cells the enzymatic reaction zones of the TPPase are normally found in the supranuclear region as a broad and caplike formation. In cases of varicocele the activity is markedly reduced, showing small areas only, while in cases of long-standing and serious varicoceles the activity is limited to a contracted globe-like plaque.

In the peritubular and interstitial Leydig cells the enzymatic activity of TPPase decreased to a varying degree. 3 β-hydroxy-Δ^5-steroid-dehydrogenase (3 β-HSDH) activity was reduced. 17 β-HSDH, alcohol dehydrogenase, etc. were found at normal intensity.

The impairment of the Sertoli cell function is correlated with the function of Leydig cell in many cases of spermatogenesis disorders.

Histomorphological and Morphometrical Studies on Intratesticular Blood Vessels

Intratesticular varicosis is histologically shown by an increase in number and by the dilatation of the venous vessels. The vascular walls become hypertrophic in the tunica media and hyalinized in the entire wall. It is too early to state whether the degree of damage is higher in the arterial or in the venous component of the capillary network. The arterioles offer resistance in order to regulate the intratesticular

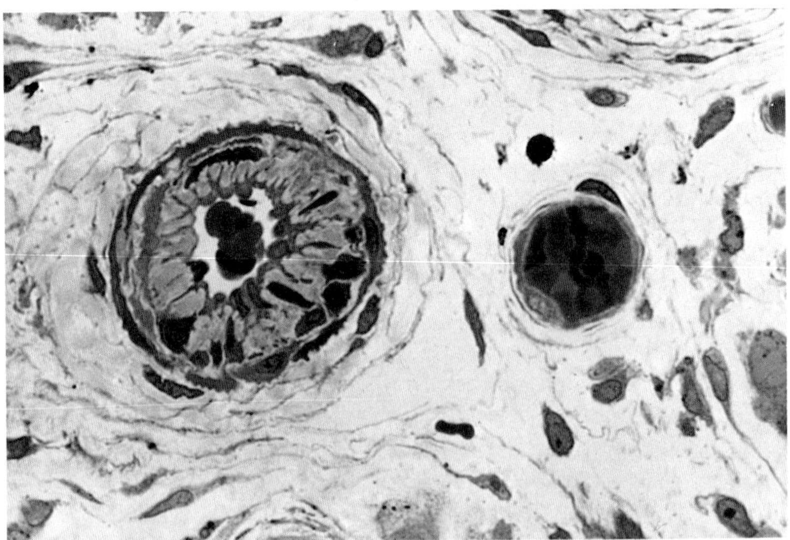

Fig. 2. Endothelial proliferation in a small testicular artery with hyalinosis of the adventitial sheath, adjacent to a dilatated venous vessel (semithin section)

Table 3. Mean diameters of arteriolar wall and lumen and ratio of diameter of the wall to the entire diameter [1]

Testicular arterioles		Varicocele II.°	Normal testis
		$n = 20$	$n = 50$
Diameter of the wall	$\overline{m}$	10.5	8.4
(µm)	s	4.6	2.6
Diameter of the lumen	$\overline{m}$	7.0	11.3
(µm)	s	1.8	4.2
Ratio of the diameter of the wall	$\overline{m}$	72.6	59.6
to the entire diameter (%)	s	12.7	9.7

blood pressure. The testicular arterioles show a hyalinization of the adventitial sheath in cases of varicocele, which has been reported by Hornstein [6], Hatakeyama et al. [2], and Suoranta [11]. The adventitial hyalinosis of the arterioles and small arterias may also be found in other testicular disorders. However, in cases of varicocele the endothelial proliferation reaches a stage (Fig. 2), which is more pronounced compared with other testicular diseases. In long-standing cases the lumen of the arterioles was even occluded. In varicocele patients unsuccessfully operated on, these morphological lesions were a general finding, suggesting a probable irreversibility of the decreased ratio of the diameter of the lumen and the thickness of the wall (Table 3).

Histological Studies on Tunica Albuginea and Mediastinum Testis

The cause of varicocele orchiopathy is an intratesticular vascular disorder. As in other venous diseases the difference of the venous pressure gradient is the causative factor provoking the pathological lesions of the vascular system and the testis parenchyma. In the opinion of the authors, the bloodstream of the renotesticular reflux may not enter the intratesticular vascular system directly and continuously, due to the extended network of peritesticular phlebostomoses. This would lead to the assumption that a double bloodstream enters the testicle, one being the normal arterial inflow and the other the pathological venous bloodstream.

In addition to the intratesticular cause of varicocele orchiopathy, the impaired function of the tunica albuginea and the mediastinum testis seems to play a decisive role. This can be concluded from the histopathological alterations of these regions. Normally the testicular venous bloodstream flows centrally to the rete and mediastinum testis. In the periphery, the veins are drained into the large veins of the septulae, which are directed to the veins of the tunica vasculosa, and through these to the mediastinum testis. This peripheral venous blood circulation shows characteristic morphological structures, which were observed on post mortem examinations:

1. Small throstle veins (Fig. 3) and arteries within the tunica vasculosa.

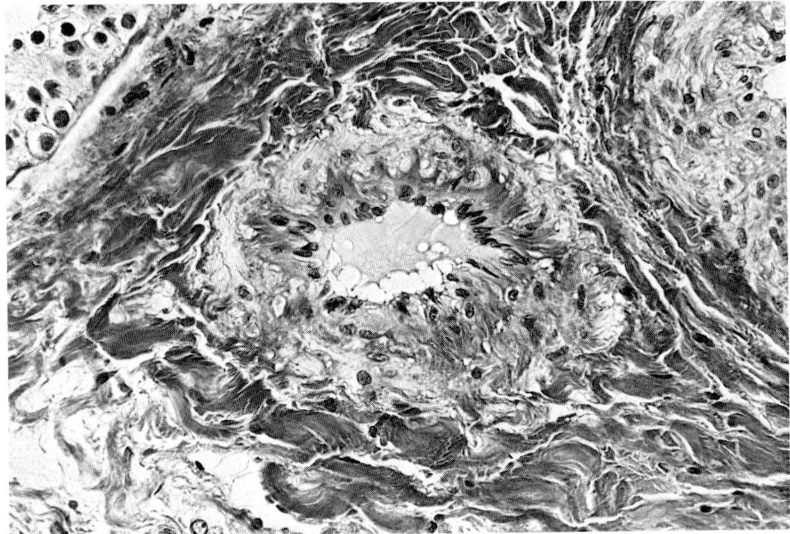

Fig. 3. Throstle vein observed in tunica vasculosa

2. Large throstle veins in the mediastinum testis.
3. An equally large arteriovenous anastomosis accompanied by a local neuroen-docrinium of nerve bundles, Leydig cells, and a Paccinian corpuscle.

Although the function of these structures is not entirely understood at present, the throstle veins and the arteriovenous shunts probably involve the contractile

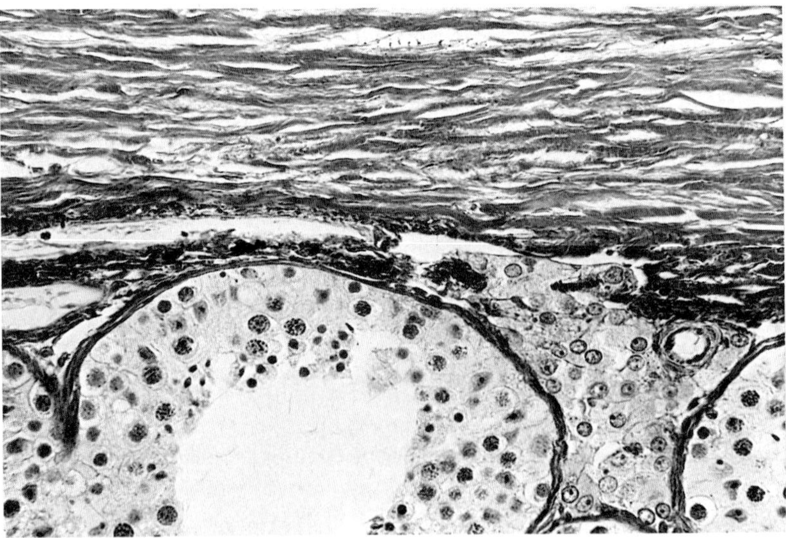

Fig. 4. Tunica vasculosa of a normal testis

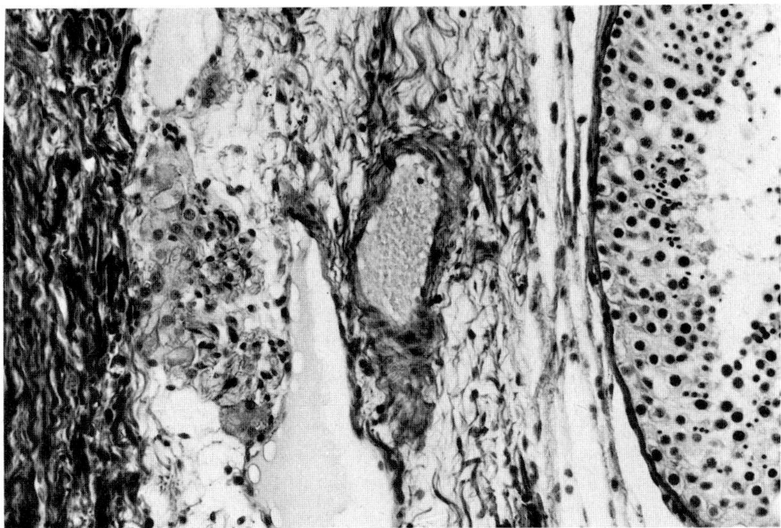

Fig. 5. Tunica vasculosa of a case of left-sided varicocele

mechanisms of the tunica albuginea, mechanisms which are essential for the outflow of tubular fluid and for the transport of spermatozoa to the vasa efferentia of the epididymis. These processes are under control of adrenergic and cholinergic nerves, and are also influenced by the Leydig cells of the mediastinum testis and the tunica albuginea. In cases of varicocele these mechanisms are impaired.

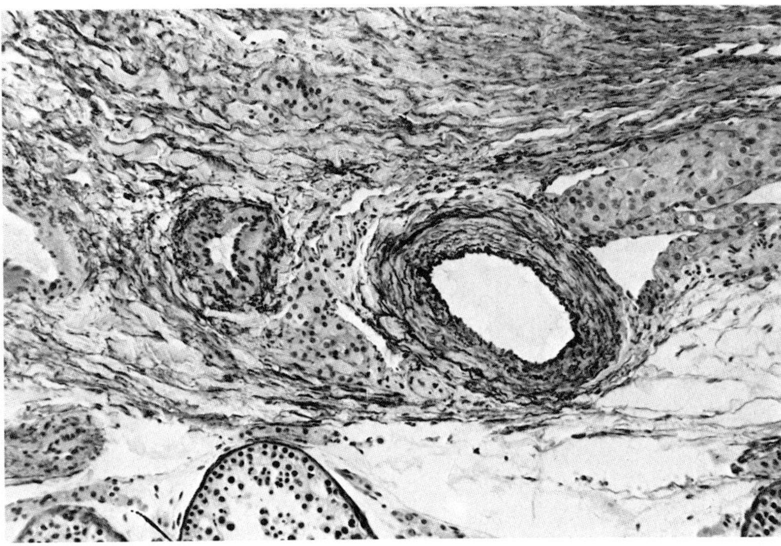

Fig. 6. Arterial, venous and lymphatic vessels, and Leydig's cell complexes in the tunica vasculosa and albuginea in a case of left-sided varicocele I/II°

The following morphological observations were made:

1. The muscle bundles of the tunica albuginea were hypertrophic.
2. Leydig cell complexes were found inside the tunica albuginea, mainly in the neighbourhood of nerves, veins, and capillaries. The veins were enlarged and the lymph capillaries were markedly dilatated.
3. The diameter of the tunica vasculosa was enlarged and the tissue exhibited edema. The number of veins were increased; the lumina were widely open. The walls of the venous blood vessels were hypertrophic and hyalinized. Also, dilatated lymph capillaries were found (Figs. 4–6). Leydig cell complexes were observed adjacent to the walls of the lymph capillaries.
4. The number of throstle veins and arteries increased considerably in cases of varicocele.

The morphological findings reported here lead the authors to suggest some compensatory mechanisms of the impaired contractile function of the tunica albuginea. The extremely dilatated lymph capillaries in the tunica vasculosa and the tunica albuginea may be regarded as morphological signs of a decompensation of this function.

References

1. Glindemann JR, Manzke HC (1980) Histologisch-morphometrische Untersuchungen zur Orthologie und Pathologie der Testes-Gefäße. Inaugural-Dissertation, Düsseldorf 1980
2. Hatakeyama S, Sengoka K, Takayama S (1966) Histological and submicroscopic studies on arteriolar hyalinosis of the human testis. Bull Tokyo Med Dent Univ 13:511–530
3. Hilscher W (1980) Zur Spermatogenese des Menschen. Therapiewoche 30:214–236
4. Hilscher B, Hofmann N, Hilscher W, Passia D, Kiesewetter D (1980) Beiträge zum Verhalten der Geschlechtszellen im basalen Compartment der Tubuli seminiferi bei fertilitätsgestörten Patienten. Veterinär-Humanmedizinische Tagung in Hannover, 21–23 February 1980. Zuchthygiene 15:96
5. Hofmann N, Kuwert E (1979) Die chronische, nicht Erreger-bedingte Orchitis. Z Hautkr 54:173–180
6. Hornstein OP (1964) Zur Klinik und Histopathologie des männlichen primären Hypogonadismus. III. Mitteilung: Hodenparenchymschäden durch Varicocelen. Arch Klin Exp Dermatol 218:347–383
7. Kiesewetter D (1980) Quantitativ-histologische Untersuchungen zur Spermatogenese fertilitätsgestörter Patienten. Inaugural-Dissertation Düsseldorf 1980
8. Passia D, Hilscher B, Goslar HG, Hilscher W, Hofmann N (1979) Thiamine pyrophosphatase – TPP-ase – a "marker enzyme" of the germ cells in the rat. Horm Metab Res 11:697–698
9. Passia D, Hilscher B, Hofmann N, Hilscher W (1980) Kombinierte quantitativ-histologische und enzymhistochemische Untersuchungen menschlichen Testisgewebes bei Varicocele. In: Fortschr Fertilitätsforsch 8, Schirren C, Mettler L, Semm K, eds, Berlin, Grosse, pp. 364–366
10. Steeno O, Knops J, Declerck L, Adimoelja A, Van De Voorle H (1976) Prevention of fertility disorders by detection and treatment of varicocele at school and college age. Andrologia 8:47–53
11. Suoranta H (1971) Changes in the small blood vessels of the adult human testis in relation to age and to some pathological conditions. Virchows Arch [Pathol Anat] 352:165–181

Varicocele and Seminal Cytology

E. W. Jᴇᴄʜᴛ, R. Mᴜ̈ʟʟᴇʀ, and E. Zɪᴇɢʟᴡᴀʟɴᴇʀ

A detrimental effect of varicocele on semen quality has been demonstrated conclusively [for review, see 4, 10], though for unexplained reasons this detrimental effect is observed only in approximately 50% of patients with varicocele [4, 10].

Like any condition which potentially impairs the gonadal functions, a varicocele, if injurious to testicular function, will bring about a reduction of sperm count and motility. In addition to this nonspecific effect on sperm number and motility, a distinct change in seminal cytology has been attributed to the influence of varicocele [2, 7]. MacLeod [7] has described an increased incidence of spermatozoa with elongated heads, which he calls "tapering forms", and of amorphous and immature sperm cells in semen. He portrayed this "stress pattern" as "a characteristic and continuing response of the testes when varicocele is present". While some investigators [2] could confirm MacLeod's findings, others [3, 6] could not and even denied [3] the very existence of tapering forms.

The contradictory observations regarding the stress pattern [2, 3, 6, 7] prompted us to evaluate our own cytologic preparations collected over the years. Seminal cytology was available from 1231 patients with reduced semen quality, in 509 of whom clinical examination had demonstrated a palpable varicocele. The patients were examined in an upright position after having been standing for 2–5 min. The patients were not asked to perform a Valsalva maneuver during the examination and no other diagnostic attempts were made to confirm the palpatory findings.

Smears for seminal cytology were left to air-dry and were stained with Giemsa. For each patient, 200 sperm cells were inspected in bright field with an oil immersion system (magnification of lens × 40, total magnification × 400). The spermatozoa were classified in 10 different categories (Table 1) and the number found for each category expressed as a percentage. While surveying the smears for spermatozoa, other cells present were taken into account and their number transformed into percentage of total spermatozoa counted. Of particular interest were immature (spermatogenic) cells as well as the "degenerative" cells described by one of us (EWJ) as characteristic for the presence of a varicocele [5]. The morphological examinations in this study were made by a single observer who did not know whether the specimen she studied was delivered by a patient with or without varicocele. The chi-square test was used for statistical analysis [9].

Our results indicate a rather small difference in the seminal cytology of patients with or without varicocele (Table 1). Although a tendency was evident toward increased percentages of abnormal forms for patients with varicocele, statistically significant differences could be secured only for the percentages of normal and

Table 1. Seminal cytology of infertile patients with and without varicocele from three different studies

	Clinical varicocele	n (infertile patients)	Anomalies of head							Anomalies of neck and midpiece		Anomalies of tail	Sperma-togenic cells [a]	Degener-ative cells [a]
			Normal	Large	Small	Tapering	Amor-phous	Double	Spheroid	Cytoplas-mic droplet	other			
This study	no	622	56.8	0.7	0.3	1.7	12.8	2.3	1.2	3.0	12.0	9.2	1.9	5.6
	yes	509	55.1	0.6	0.3	1.9	15.0	2.2	1.0	2.3	11.6	10.2	2.4	7.2
								(Bicephalic)						(Immature forms)
MacLeod (7)	no	1500	57.2	5.2	10.2	12.8	12.8	1.6	–	–	–	–	4.0	–
	yes	146	34.0	5.0	10.0	23.0	25.0	3.0	–	–	–	–	16.0	–
							(Irregular)		(Conical)					
Czyglik et al. (2)	no	20	42.1	1.6	13.5	8.7	5.7	1.1	3.0	9.0	11.0	12.5	–	–
	yes	50	30.9	1.4	11.5	20.8	7.9	2.7	7.4	14.7	14.8	10.6	–	–

[a] Computed as percentage of the total number of cells of the germinal line

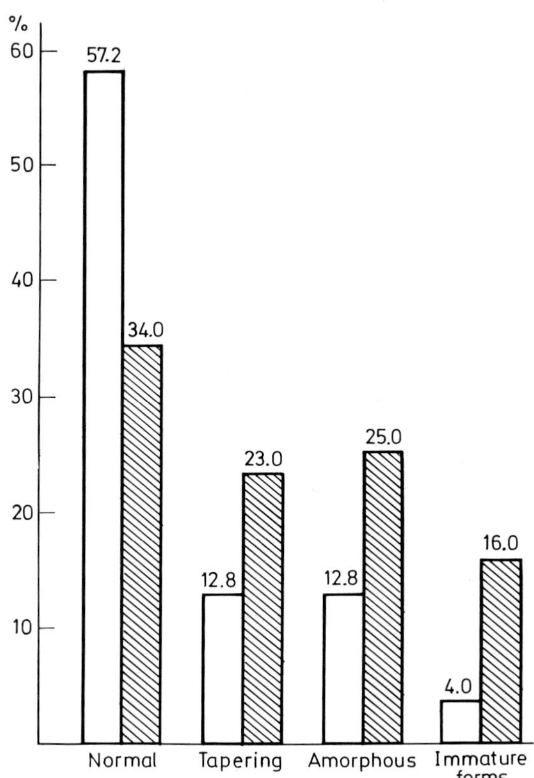

Fig. 1. Selected seminal cytology from infertile patients with (shaded columns) and without (blank columns) varicocele [7, cf. Table 1]

amorphous spermatozoa ($P < 0.01$ and < 0.001, respectively). There was, however, a statistically significant difference for the spermatogenic cells ($P < 0.01$) as well as for the degenerative cells ($P < 0.001$). The incidence of tapering forms was very small and almost equal in both patients with and without varicocele.

The proposition of a pronounced stress pattern in patients with varicocele is supported only in part by our results: we cannot confirm the pivotal role of tapering forms seen as a cornerstone in the seminal cytology of the stress pattern by MacLeod [7]. It is worth noting that even our statistically significant differences between patients with and without varicocele are much smaller than those reported by MacLeod [7] and by Czyglik et al. [2]. To demonstrate this dissimilarity, we have shown graphically the results with the largest differences for MacLeod [7], for Czyglik et al. [2], and for our data (Figs. 1–3). These graphic presentations also emphasize the almost identical percentages of tapering forms found by MacLeod [3] and Czyglik et al. [2]. Lindholmer et al. [6], on the other hand, reported an incidence of tapering forms similar – though somewhat higher – to that seen by us. Unfortunately, their data are not sufficiently detailed for a graphic presentation.

We cannot explain the conflicting results, particularly with regard to the prevalence of tapering forms. It is conceivable that MacLeod [7] as well als Czyglik et al. [2] were aware of the source of the semen they were investigating, i.e., a patient with varicocele. In the present study – as in the one published by Lindholmer et al. [6] –, the evaluation of smears was made on a single-blind basis.

The disagreement between the different investigators may also be caused by the difficult identification of tapering forms. To the best of our knowledge, no photographs of this spermatozoan form have been published by MacLeod. His schematic drawing [8], however, appears – to us – extremely artificial; we have yet to encounter a single sperm that could qualify as "tapering" when judged strictly according to this picture.

One conclusion of this study, therefore, has to be a call for a standardization of sperm morphology based on photographs of spermatozoa (de)formed typically as well as of spermatogenic and degenerative cells. The latter should, we believe, be integrated into the stress pattern. They are, in our hands, a relatively reliable – though by no means pathognomonic – indicator for the presence of a varicocele [5]. These cells and fragments of cells probably mirror the increased rate of exfoliation in the seminiferous tubules and accessory glands and of decay during the epididymal transit due to varicocele.

In conclusion, our overall results confirm the stress pattern stipulated by MacLeod [7, 8] for seminal cytology in the presence of a varicocele. They do not, however, corroborate the main feature of the stress pattern, the tapering forms. We found a relatively small incidence of tapering forms, which was almost identical for

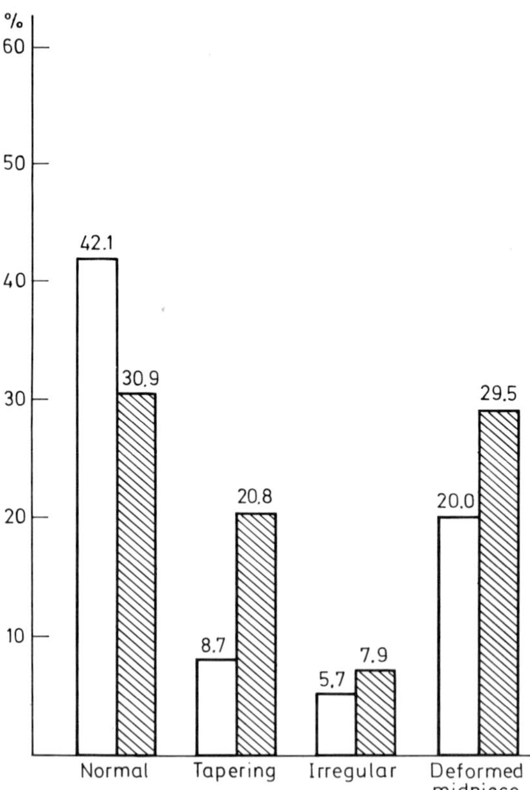

Fig. 2. Selected seminal cytology from infertile patients with (shaded columns) and without (blank columns) varicocele [2, cf. Table 1]

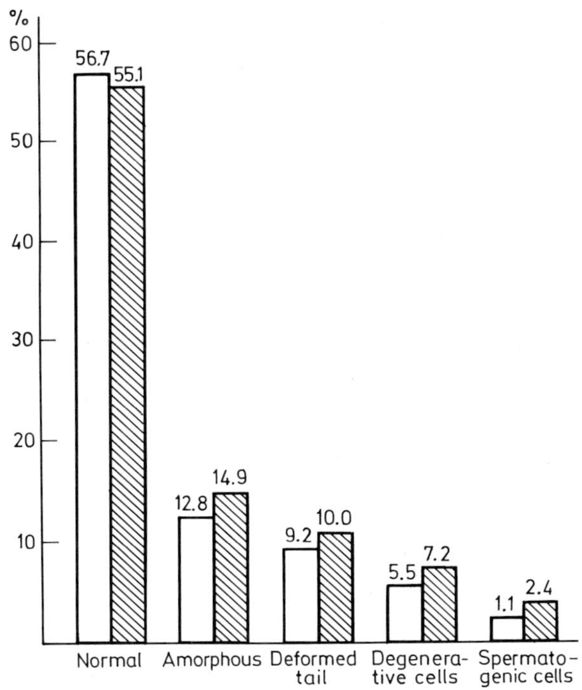

Fig. 3. Selected seminal cytology from infertile patients with (shaded columns) and without (blank columns) varicocele (this study, cf. Table 1)

patients with and without varicocele. On the other hand, our assumption regarding the significance of degenerative cells [5] was strengthened: They were seen more frequently in the semen of patients with varicocele.

Our results indicate that the analysis of seminal cytology can help but little in the detection of a subclinical [10] varicocele. The rather small differences between the seminal cytology of patients with and without varicocele, however, may permit the confirmation of a varicocele found by the Doppler technique, thermography, or retrograde phlebography (see this symposium). Finally, the evaluation of seminal cytology appears useful for controlling the effect of high ligation as pointed out previously by MacLeod [7, 8]. According to our results (see this symposium), the degenerative cells reflect particularly well the influence of percutaneous sclerosis (and of high ligation, unpublished data).

References

1. Comhaire F, Monteyne R, Kunnen M (1976) The value of scrotal thermography as compared with selective retrograde venography of the internal spermatic vein for the diagnosis of "subclinical" varicocele. Fertil Steril 27:694
2. Czyglik F, David G, Bisson JP, Jouannet P, Gernigon Cl (1973) La tératospermie du varicocèle. Nouv Presse Med 2:1127
3. Guillon G, Milhiet H (1976) Effets du traitement des varicocèles sur la stérilité masculine. Devenir de la fertilité de 84 patients opérés. Nouv Presse Med 5:2079
4. Jecht E (1977) Varikozele und Fertilität. Z Haut Geschlechtskr 138:177

 5. Jecht E (1978) Indikationen zur hohen Ligatur der Vena spermatica interna aus der Sicht des dermatologischen Andrologen. Therapiewoche 28:1905
 6. Lindholmer C, Thulin L, Eliasson R (1975) Semen characteristics before and after ligation of the left internal spermatic veins in men with varicocele. Scand J Urol Nephrol 9:177
 7. MacLeod J (1965) Seminal cytology in the presence of varicocele. Fertil Steril 16:735
 8. MacLeod J (1969) Further observations on the role of varicocele in human male fertility. Fertil Steril 20:545
 9. Siegel S (1956) Nonparametric statistics for the behavioral sciences. McGraw-Hill, New York Toronto London
10. Verstoppen GR, Steeno OP (1977) Varicocele and the pathogenesis of the associated subfertility. A review of the various theories. II. Results of surgery. Andrologia 9:293

Cases Illustrating the Variation of Results

H. Kasseckert and W. Adam

Although consideration of the clinical relevance of symptoms and the appropriateness of various forms of therapy must comply with statistical criteria, the success of therapy in individual cases cannot be predicted on such criteria alone. This paper therefore presents cases which are intended to document the inhomogeneity of ejaculate quality prior to and after therapy of so-called idiopathic varicoceles.

Case I. Normozoospermia with markedly advanced varicocele on the left side. Konstantin D., 21 years, student. Normosemia; sperm density, 60 million per milliliter; total and progressive motility, 80% and 60%; normal morphology, 69%.

Case II. Normozoospermia with markedly advanced varicocele on the left side, isolated asthenozoospermia with varicocele recurrence following high ligation. Reinhart MT., 30 years, secondary school teacher. At the initial examination pregnancy had been desired for more than 1 year. Sperm density, morphology, and motility (total, 80%; progressive, 60%) were within the normal range. Recurrence of the varicocele appeared 4 months after the high ligation, at which time total motility was 60% and progressive motility, 20%. After another 7 months total motility was 40%; other parameters were unchanged.

Case III. Normalization of all ejaculate parameters following high ligation of markedly advanced varicocele on the left side and subsequent formation of a hydrocele testis on the left side. Ali K., age 31 years, laborer. At the initial examination pregnancy had been desired for more than 2½ years. An epididymidal infiltration was detectable, which could not be verified clinically in later examination. Sperm density was 1.65 million per milliliter (total 4.125 million); total motility, 50%; progressive motility, 30%; normal morphology, 52%. High ligation was performed 2 years after the initial examination. All parameters were normal 4–6 months postoperatively (sperm density, 81–115 million per milliliter; total motility, 80%; progressive motility, 60–70%) despite development of a hydrocele in the interim. Patient's spouse did not become pregnant. Polyzoospermia (336 million per milliliter, reduced total motility) appeared 20 months after the hydrocele operation (performed 8 months after high ligation).

Case IV. Distinct improvement of progressive oligoastheno-teratozoospermia following high bilateral ligation of bilateral varicoceles. Uwe H., 37 years, engineer. In May 1978 sperm density was 15 million per milliliter and subsequently fell to 2 million per ml (8 million total) under outside treatment with kallikrein/mesterolone followed by HMG/mesterolone. Normal morphology was 40%; total and progressive motility, 20% and 10% respectively. Anamnesis did not provide an explanation for the deterioration. Clinical examination showed testes with reduced tonus and normal volume. Three months after surgery, the varicocele was reduced on the right side and no longer detectable on the left side; histology revealed a second degree maturation arrest on the left side. Sperm density was 32 million per milliliter (total 128 million); total and progressive motility, 70% and 50% respectively; and normal morphology, 50%.

Case V. Oligoastheno-teratozoospermia with testes bordering on atrophy and varicocele on the left side. High ligation without subsequent improvement of ejaculate quality. Spousal pregnancy at the time of the operation. Walter B., 30 Years, assistant lawyer. Apart from moderate nicotine consumption there were no fertility-reducing causal factors. Both testes measured approximately 12 ml. Nicotine abstinence and kallikrein did not yield ejaculate with only normal parameters, but occasionally individual parameters were only slightly impaired (sperm density, 8.5–3.20 million per milliliter; total motility, 30–80%; progressive motility, 10–60%, normal morphology, 37–64%). Fractionation did not yield substantial improvement in quality. Spousal conception occurred directly before high ligation. Five months after surgery, ejaculate parameters were not improved. Palpation did not indicate recurrence of the varicocele.

Case VI. Improvement of an oligoasthenozoospermia with varicocele on the left side, spousal conception directly following high ligation.

Mehmet K., 23 years. Pregnancy had been desired for more than 2 years. Sperm density increased from 25.2 to 42 million per milliliter 4 months after the operation. Total motility improved from 60 to 70% and progressive motility from 0 to 20%. Spousal conception occurred directly after release from clinical treatment.

Markedly advanced varicoceles can also be accompanied by normal ejaculate quality – according to the accepted parameters for judging fertility. In one of the six demonstrated cases the initially normal parameters actually deteriorated significantly after therapy and recidivation. At least for a certain time, however, dramatic inprovement or normalization of parameters occurred in two cases, one of which involved time- and cost-intensive attempts at medical therapy.

Another remarkable feature of these six cases is that the spouses of 2 patients became pregnant near the time of the surgery. In one case, conception was not very probable in light of the preoperative development, and in the other case, conception could hardly have been due to the effect of surgery.

III. Diagnosis

A. Phlebography

Technique of Retrograde Phlebography of the Internal Spermatic Vein

W. Seyferth, E. I. Richter, and R. Grosse-Vorholt

A radiological statement on an angiographic examination technique includes a view on the equipment and on the radiation exposure of the patient who undergoes a primary diagnostic procedure, and a description of the catheter technique applied and the results obtained.

The examination is performed on a tilting X-ray table under a fluoroscopic apparatus with TV image intensifier photography. Single shots with a picture frequency of one per second are usually sufficient for phlebographic examination procedures. The medium screening time is about 90 s for demonstrating the left spermatic vein. Demonstration of the right spermatic vein, with its much more complicated examination technique, however, requires 200 s.

If the scanning field constantly covers approximately 100 cm² during the sounding period, the admitted radiation dose is 1.5 rad on the left side and 3.5 rad on the right. The total radiation exposure is approximately 5 rad. The mathematically calculated gonadal load is 400 mrad. The testes of the patient are protected with caps and fluoroscopy is carried out only up to the terminal line.

The aim of a phlebographic examination procedure is to furnish the highest possible number of selective demonstrations of the internal spermatic vein on both sides with the lowest possible risk for the patient.

Subsequent to the ascertainment of the history, the right femoral vein can be punctured under local anesthesia without further premedication. The puncture itself is carried out at the patient's middle breathing activity to avoid a Gullmo femoral compression phenomenon. When advancing the needle, a slight aspiration through a record syringe, half-filled with salt solution, is favorable.

In selecting the catheter type, which now must be introduced over a guide wire with flexible tip under TV image intensifier fluoroscopy, one must note that in nearly 100% of cases the left spermatic vein opens into the left renal vein, whereas in about 90% of cases the right spermatic vein opens into the inferior caval vein and only in 10% into the renal vein [1]. Only the specific selective location of the catheter in the spermatic vein will furnish good information on the grade of insufficiency.

The examination begins on the left side of the spermatic vein. Because of the varying distance between the orifice of the spermatic vein and the renal vein, we use catheters (fig. 1) specially made for selective phlebography; these differ by the varying length of the last angled catheter section but one.

First, the catheter tip must be located in the renal vein as near as possible to the kidney. Then follows application of contrast material, withdrawing the catheter step by step, each time under the patient's forceful Valsalva maneuver. When the end of

Fig. 1. Catheter for demonstrating the internal spermatic vein (from left to right): right Sidewinder II; and special left catheters with different lengths of the last but one catheter section

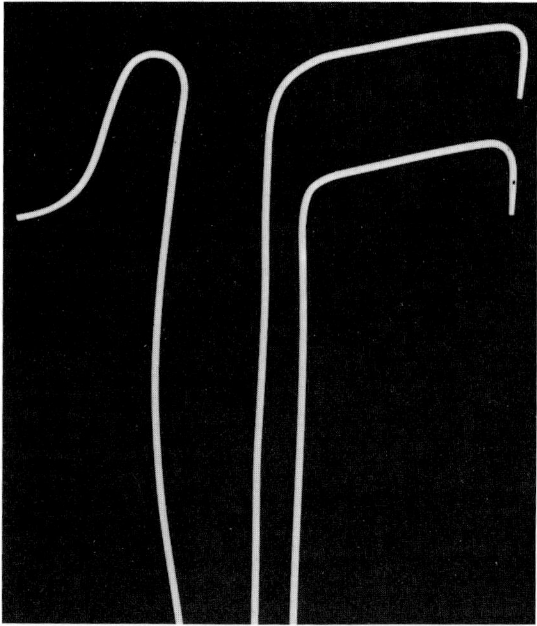

the spermatic vein is contrast-filled, selective examination of the vessel can be tried (Fig. 2).

The statement "insufficiency of the spermatic vein" is possible only after thorough control of the renal vein from its periphery to the caval vein. A contrast-filled renal vein delivering a panoramic picture does not suffice.

First, pragmatic reasons led us to classify an insufficiency of the spermatic vein at selective positioning of the catheter into three stages, as follows: [5]

Insufficiency stage I
– contrast material column longer than 5 cm from the insufficient valve.

Insufficiency stage II
– contrast material column up to the fourth/fifth lumbar vertebral body.

Insufficiency stage III
– contrast material column exceeding the iliac crest down to the scrotum.

Correlation of these classifications to clinical parameters is still pending. For the moment, however, a description of the results obtained with sclerotherapy might be helpful. Demonstration of the right spermatic vein, however, is much more complicated because of its inconstant location, and above all because of its marked angulation as it leaves the inferior caval vein.

According to the information in the available literature, the percentages of proved varicoceles on the right side vary between 5% and 20% [3, 4].

We started searching for the orifice of the right spermatic vein into the infrarenal caval vein with a catheter normally used for the left spermatic vein. Here, however, the first curved catheter section acted like a tension spring on the left wall of the caval vein when starting from the right. This is favorable for demonstrating the opening of the spermatic vein (Fig. 3). Often, however, a sufficient selective location of this catheter in the right spermatic vein fails and reliable information on the real stage of insufficiency cannot be obtained. If the orifice of the spermatic vein cannot be found in the wall of the caval vein, the right renal vein must be explored with the same catheter and in the same way as on the left side.

When the orifice has been found, the catheter must be exchanged with a normal Sidewinder II (Fig. 1). The catheter tip must then be advanced on the guide wire; in this way a selective introduction of the catheter into the right spermatic vein is nearly always successful. Assessment of the real extent of the varicocele is subsequently possible (Fig. 4). Often, however, the Sidewinder tip catches in the orifice of the spermatic vein into the right renal vein. Depending on the distance between the orifice and the caval vein, we use the short-arched catheter that Bigot [2] recommends, and sometimes the left-sided catheter for coronary angiography.

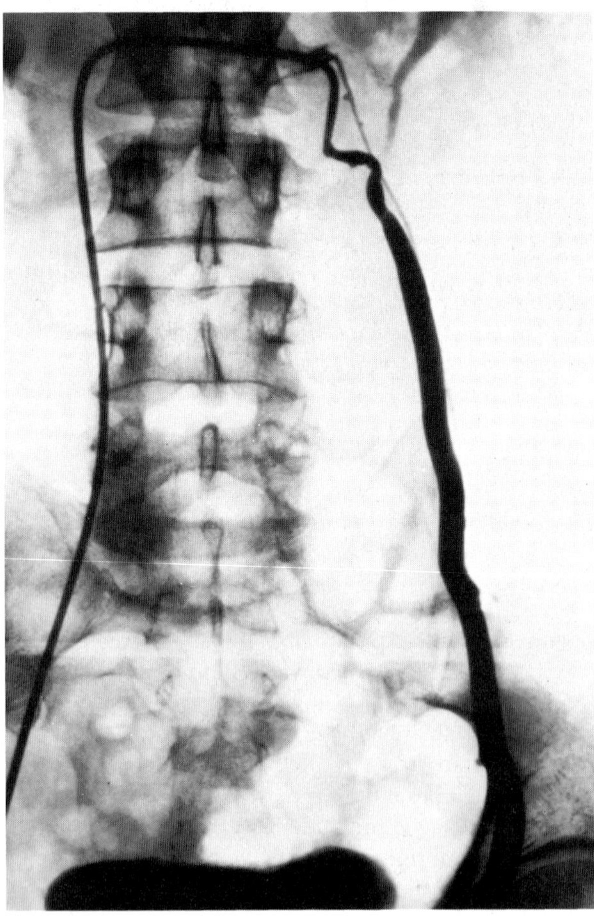

Fig. 2. Varicocele, left, stage III

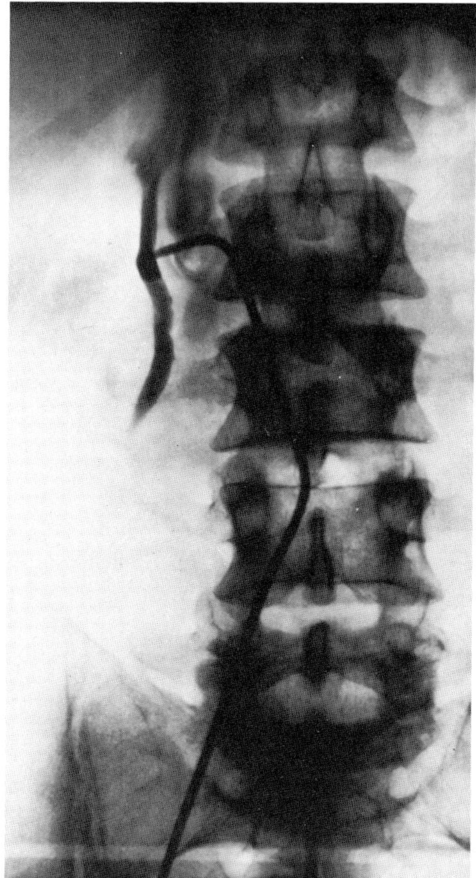

Fig. 3. Sounding, right

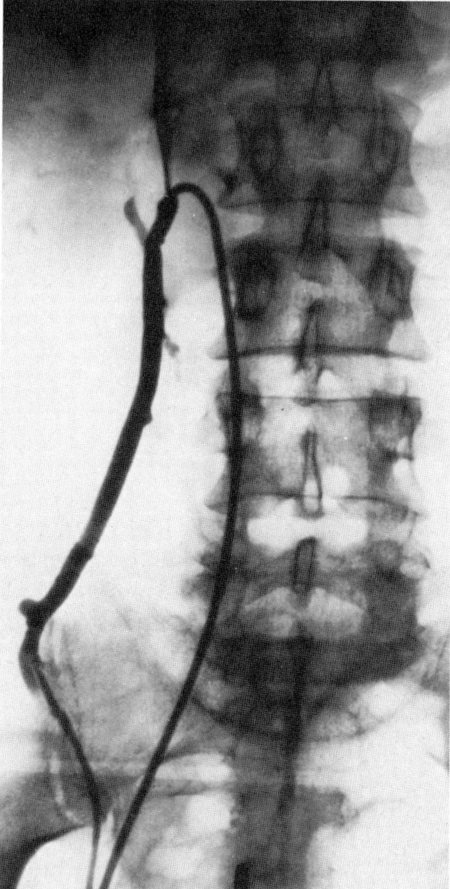

Fig. 4. Selective demonstration (varicocele stage III)

An analysis of the examination data obtained with the new technique will prove the efficiency of the new method.

We found in 68.5% of 419 patients a varicocele on the left side, and in 13.6% on the right side. In the same examination procedure, we performed sclerotherapy in 164 cases, 12 on the right and 152 on the left side.

On analysis of the examination data we found that – always using the same catheter types – experience has an influence on the result which can be obtained with sclerotherapy in the left spermatic vein, whereas in the right spermatic vein not only does experience play an important role but even more decisive is the modified examination technique. In this connection we stated an increase of the success rate from 64% to 73% on the left side, but from 5.1% to 19.5% on the right side (Table 1).

In the last examination group we found a success rate of 90% on the left and a little less than 60% on the right side. However, these precentages should be regarded cautiously since a success rate of 90% cannot always be expected on the left side.

Table 1. Influence of experience and catheter-procedure development on success rates of varicoceles

Side	Cases 0 – 292 (n = 292)	Cases 293 – 375 (n = 82)	Cases 376 – 419 (n = 44)
Left	187 (64.0%)	60 (73.2%)	40 (90.9%)
Right	15 (5.1%)	16 (19.5%)	26 (59.1%)

Table 2. Influence of experience on success rates in sclerotherapy

Side	Cases 0 – 132 (n = 132)	Cases 133 – 164 (n = 32)	Total (n = 164)
Right	2 (1.5%)	10 (31.3%)	12
Left	130 (98.5%)	22 (68.7%)	152

A look at the classification of sclerotherapies (Table 2) is also informative. Of the first 132 sclerotherapies, only 2 were performed on the right side. In the last examination group in which the modified technique was applied, 10 sclerotherapies were performed on the right side versus 22 on the left.

A successful outcome of the sclerotherapy can only be expected at selective location of the catheter in the internal spermatic vein. In the first 375 examined cases we found 31 varicoceles on the right side; 2 of them (6.5%) were successfully sclerosed. The ratio on the left side, however, was 247:130 (52.6%). In the last 44 cases examined 26 varicoceles were proved on the right side. Ten of them were sclerosed. This means an increase to 38.5%, whereas 22 of 40 varicoceles on the left side were sclerosed, i.e., 55%.

One may conclude from these results that the improved examination technique did not yield a considerably better success rate on the left side, but did on the right. This stimulates again the discussion on the frequency of varicoceles on the right side and their phlebographic manifestations.

In our case studies of primary male infertility and pathological spermatogram, varicoceles on the right side, discovered with the new examination technique, seem to be more frequent than has been so far presumed. The percentages we found are considerably higher than those reported in the literature to date.

References

1. Ahlberg NE, Bartheley O, Chidakel N, Fritjiofsson A (1966) Phlebography in varicocele scroti. Acta Radiol [Diagn] (Stockh) 4:517
2. Bigot JM, Chatel A, Dectot H, Hélénon CH (1978) La phlébographie spermatique retrograde. – Interêt dans la varicocèle. Dept. de Radiodiagnostic de l'Hôpital Tenon, Paris
3. Iaccarino V (1977) Trattamento conservativo del varicocele: Flebografia selettiva e scleroterapia delle vene gonadiche. Riv Radiol 17:107
4. Riedl P (1979) Selektive Phlebographie und Katheter-Thrombosierung der Vena testicularis bei primärer Varicocele. Wien Med Wochenschr [Suppl] 91:99
5. Zeitler E, Jecht E, Richter EI, Seyferth W (1979) Technik und Ergebnisse der Spermatika-Phlebographie bei 136 Männern mit primärer Sterilität. ROEFO 131:179

Radiologic Anatomy of the Left Testicular Vein in Varicoceles

P. RIEDL

Depending on the technique adopted, surgery for varicoceles involving the left testicular vein is associated with a postoperative persistence rate of 1%–20% [4, 9, 16, 18, 24]. In most cases, failure to ligate single venous branches or collaterals bypassing a functional ligation are responsible for varicocele persistence [14]. Except for the studies by Chatel et al. [6, 7], the nature and number of left testicular vein branches are poorly documented [5, 8, 10, 11, 14, 15].

In 1979 the radiologic anatomy of the vein was described on the basis of 67 cases. The present contribution is a synopsis of these and includes a number of cases examined subsequently.

Material and Method

A total of 137 patients with leftsided varicoceles, aged between 13 and 48 years, underwent phlebography. In 14 cases the selective renal technique was employed [1, 2]; in 9 cases a vein of the pampiniform plexus was exposed and selective angiography was done in an antegrade fashion; and in 114 patients selective retrograde venography following the abnormal blood stream was used [6–8, 14, 21, 23, 25, 27]. The patients were additionally subjected to intraoperative phlebography [5, 10, 12, 17].

While serial angiograms were recorded in the first 18 cases, no more than 2 to 3 films were exposed as directed by fluoroscopy in the remaining patients (for each film, 10–15 cc of the radiopaque substance was injected manually). If the vein failed to fill adequately with the patient reclining, additional films were recorded with the patient standing (Valsalva maneuver). Figure 1 shows a diagram of the left testicular vein with the vascular structures evaluated in all patients.

Results

Inadequate visualization of some venous segments (e.g., the renal vein on selective testicular vein filling, the infra-inguinal anastomoses on shielding the inguinal region, or for other mostly technical reasons) ruled out an accurate assessment of the parameters chosen in some of the 137 cases.

The entry of the testicular vein into the renal vein was found to be remarkably constant. It was consistently located within a segment of 3 cm; in about half of the

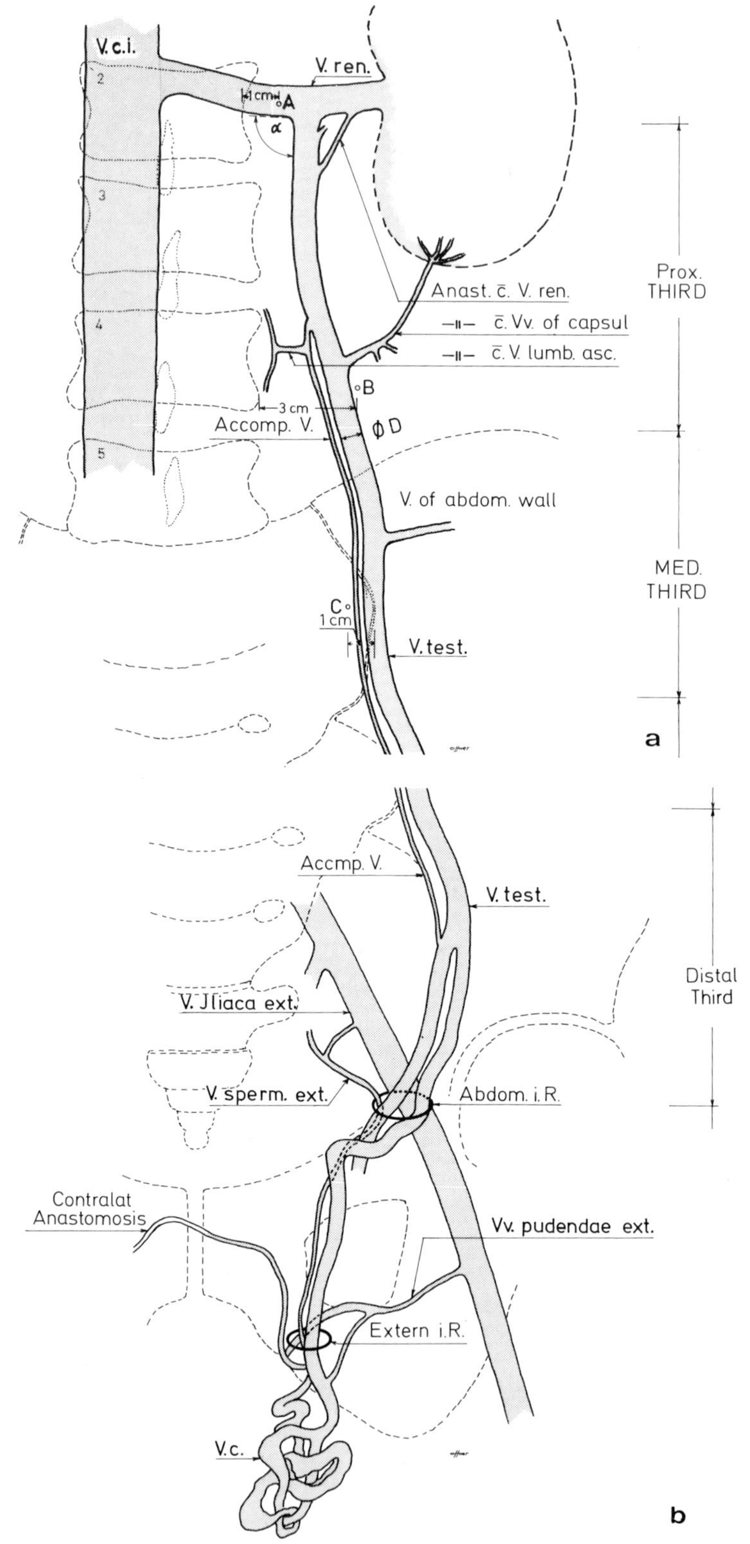

V. c. i.
V. ren.
1 cm
A
α
2
3
4
5
Anast. c̄. V. ren.
—ıı— c̄. Vv. of capsul
—ıı— c̄. V. lumb. asc.
B
3 cm
ØD
Accomp. V.
V. of abdom. wall
C
1 cm
V. test.
Prox.
THIRD
MED.
THIRD
a
Accmp. V.
V. test.
V. Jliaca ext.
V. sperm. ext.
Abdom. i. R.
Contralat
Anastomosis
Vv. pudendae ext.
Extern i. R.
V. c.
Distal
Third
b

Table 1. Course of left renal vein in 89 patients with left-sided varicocele

Renal vein	n	%	
Horizontal	31	34.8	
Ascending towards inferior v. cava	37	41.6	} 76.4
Descending towards inferior v. cava	8	9.0	
Two renal veins	13	14.6	} 23.6
Total	89	100.0	

Table 2. Morphology of testicular vein valves

Testicular vein valves	n	%
Absent	114	83.2
Residual incompetent valves	18	13.1
Competent valves bypassed by collaterals	5	3.7
Total	137	100.0

cases within a segment of no more than 1 cm (measured from a fictitious point A located 1 cm left of the lumbar spine; see Fig. 1). In 10% of cases with dense paralumbar venous plexuses the point of entry was not unequivocally identifiable. The course and number of renal veins are shown in Table 1. The angle between the testicular and renal veins was obtuse (95°–120°) in about half of the evaluable cases and acute (60°–85°) in about one-sixth; in about a third of the patients the testicular vein entered the renal vein at a right angle (85°–95°).

On selective retrograde filling the testicular vein diameter was found to measure 4–12 mm (mean, 7.01 ± 2.13 mm) and to be proportionate to the size of the varicocele (the difference of testicular vein diameters in varicoceles grade I versus those of grades II and III was statistically significant at $P < 0.05$). Valves were absent in 114 instances (83.2%); in 18 cases (13.1%) residual incompetent valves were present; and in 5 cases (3.7%) competent valves were bypassed by collaterals (Table 2, Fig. 2).

Unlike the entry into the renal vein, the course of the testicular vein showed considerable variation. In fact, the vein was found to course within 2.5 cm of two fictitious points B and C left of the spine (Fig. 1). The closer the vein came to the lumbar spine, the more numerous were the anastomoses (Fig. 3).

In Tables 3–6, the emphasis is on the presence of venous branches rather than on their number and caliber. (The diameter of accompanying veins was arbitrarily limited to 2 mm; vessels with a caliber in excess of 2 mm were considered as double

Fig. 1 a, b. Diagram showing the site of entry and the angle between the left testicular and the renal veins as well as the supra- and infrainguinal anastomoses

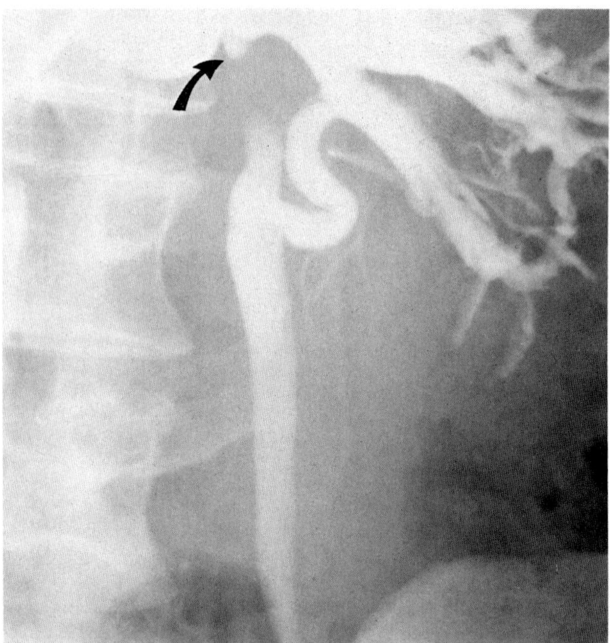

Fig. 2. Selective renal vein phlebography. Competent valve in the proximal testicular vein (↗). Collateral bypassing the valve with adequate filling of distal testicular vein (diameter = 10 mm) and extensive varicocele

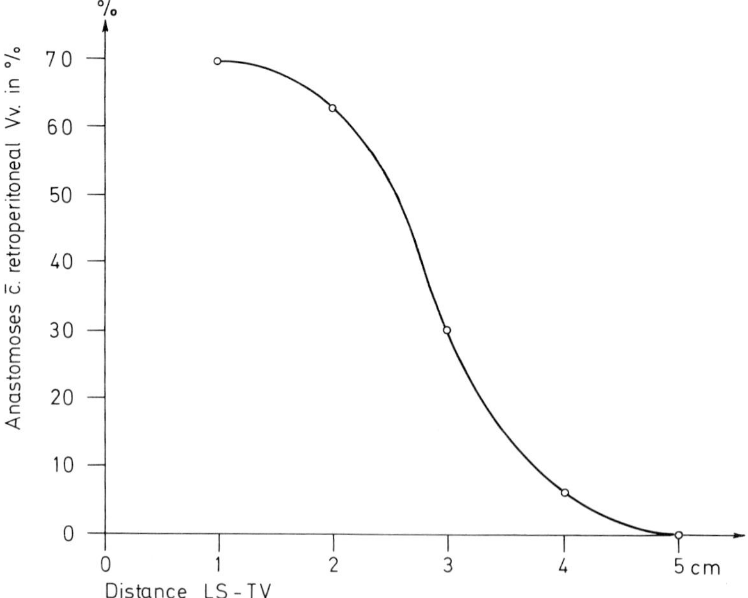

Fig. 3. Number of anastomoses with paralumbar veins relative to the distance of the testicular vein from the left border of the spinal column

Table 3. Frequency of supra- and infrainguinal anastomoses of the left testicular vein

Testicular vein anastomoses	Present		Absent		Could not be evaluated	
Supra-inguinal	n	%	n	%	n	%
With renal vein	71	51.8	40	29.2	26	19.0
With capsular and ureteric veins	75	54.7	32	23.4	30	21.9
With renal and/or capsular veins	108	78.8	22	16.1	7	5.1
With paralumbar veins	96	70.1	36	26.3	5	3.6
With abdominal wall veins	50	36.5	81	59.1	6	4.4
Proximal third	126	92.0	11	8.0		
Middle third	111	81.0	26	19.0		
Distal third	81	59.1	56	40.0		
Infrainguinal (draining the serotum, $n = 58$)						
Homolateral	43	74.1	15	25.9		
Contralateral	24	41.4	34	58.6		

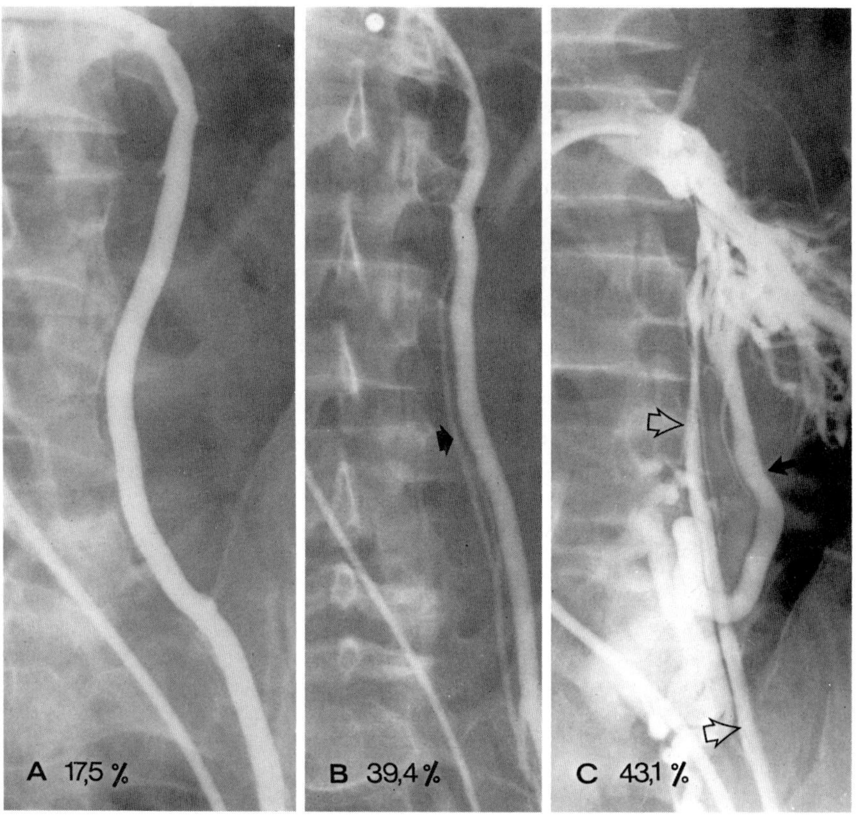

Fig. 4a–c. Anatomical variants of left testicular vein: **a** collaterals absent; **b** accompanying vessel (→); **c** testicular vein (⇉) with numerous anastomoses ⬅ (see text)

veins.) A clear differentiation of suprainguinal anastomoses by communications with the renal and the capsular veins was not feasible in all cases so that these anastomoses were listed en bloc (Table 3).

In view of their implications for surgery, all collaterals were evaluated relative to the level of the testicular vein. Collaterals were found to be much more common in

Table 4. Number of venous channels (diameter < 2 mm) accompanying the left testicular vein

Accompanying vein	n	%
Absent	60	43.8
1	49	35.8
2	16	11.7
> 2 (venous plexus)	12	8.7
Total	137	100.0

Table 5. Morphology of main left testicular vein

		n	%
Divisions of testicular vein		76	55.5
5 cm suprainguinal	22		
< 10 cm suprainguinal	12	45	32.8
< 20 cm suprainguinal	11		
Paralumbar venous plexus		11	8.1
Two veins		5	3.6
Total		137	100.0

Table 6. Number of venous vessels within the area drained by the left internal testicular vein at the level of the internal inguinalring

Number of veins	n	%	
1	16	11.7	
2	28	20.4	
3	49	35.8	
4	27	19.7	75.8
5	3	2.2	
6 and more	1	0.7	
not evaluable	13	9.5	
Total	137	100.0	

the proximal two-thirds versus the distal third. Communications to the deep leg and pelvic veins (about 30%) almost always originated in the infrainguinal region. Wide suprainguinal anastomoses were found in only 6 cases. Accompanying veins and venous plexuses were present in more than 50% of cases (Table 4).

Approximately 50% of the patients showed suprainguinal divisions, plexuses, or two distinct vessels (Table 5), while at the level of the internal inguinal ring more than one distinct vessels (Table 6) was noted in over 80% of cases.

Three variant patterns were distinguished:

Type A (n = 24, 17.5%):
A single, distinct testicular vein without lateral branches, but with fine ramifications in the proximal third.

Type B (n = 54, 39.4%):
A distinct testicular vein accompanied by several parallel venous channels (maximum diameter 2 mm); fine ramifications may be present in the proximal third.

Type C (n = 59, 43.10%):
Numerous branches along the entire course of the vein (Fig. 4).

Discussion

While the course, anastomoses, branching pattern, etc. of the testicular vein show considerable variability, the entry into the renal vein is remarkably constant. On an average, it comes to lie about 1 cm left of the second lumbar vertebral body. As a consequence, selective filling is unproblematic and, since the fluorscopy time is short (less than 2 min on an average), the radiation dose delivered is low. The number of the left renal veins present and their course were felt to be of particular interest, as anatomical studies showed preaortic renal veins to ascend towards the inferior vena cava, while retroaortic renal veins descend towards the inferior vena cava [3, 13, 19, 20]. If doubled, the left renal vein forms a renal collar encircling the aortic in more than 99% of cases [3, 19, 20]. Using these morphological criteria, which can be verified by ultrasound [22], about 25% of our cases had retroaortic renal veins and venous rings. This contrast with a reported occurrence of about 9% to 16% [13, 19, 26] in the literature.

Aside from the compression of the preaortic renal vein between the abdominal aorta and the superior mesenteric artery, the unfavourable angle between the tes-

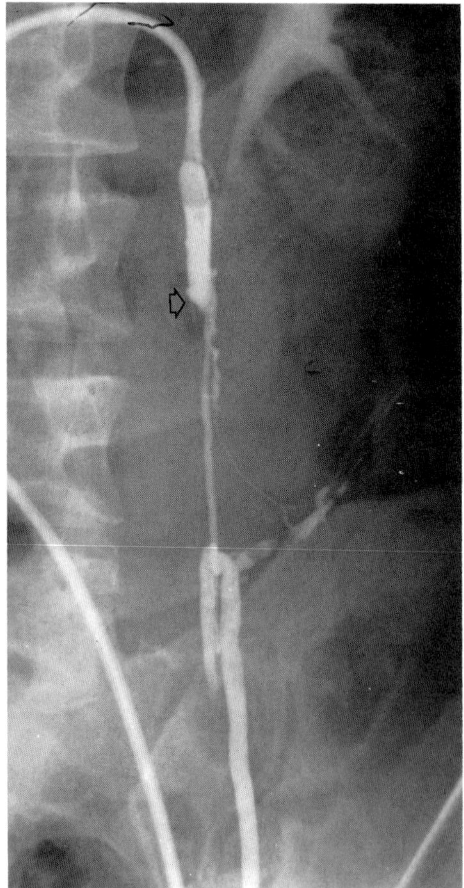

Fig. 5. Postoperative persistence of varicocele after infrarenal ligation and establishment of collateral circulation

ticular vein and left renal vein, and the more common congenital absence of valves on the left side [19], this might well be one factor explaining why more than 90% of all varicoceles are located on the left side.

The nature, number, and course of retroperitoneal anastomoses are of prime importance for treatment. This implies that, in the absence of preoperative phlebography, surgery should be confined to suprainguinal ligation just above the internal inguinal ring. Unless all venous channels in this region (5–6 at most) are meticulously dissected, surgery is unlikely to keep the rate of postoperative varicocele persistence under 1% (4, 9). Anastomoses and accompanying venous channels above this level are difficult to identify intraoperatively and may be responsible for postoperatively persisting varicoceles (Fig. 5).

Summary

On the basis of 137 selective left testicular vein phlebographies in patients with varicocele the anatomy of the vessel is reviewed and implications of its anatomy for surgical treatment are discussed.

References

1. Ahlberg NE, Bartley O, Chidekel N (1965) Retrograde contrast filling of the left gonadal vein. Acta Radiol 3:385
2. Ahlberg NE, Bartley O, Chidekel N, Fritjofsson A (1966) Phlebography in varicocele scroti. Acta Radiol 4:517
3. Anson BJ, Cauldwell EW, Pick JW, Beaton LE (1974) The blood supply of the kidney, suprarenal gland and associated structures. Surg Gynecol Obstet 84:313
4. Brown JS (1976) Varicocelectomy in the subfertile male: A tenyear experience with 295 cases. Fertil Steril 27:1046
5. Brown JS, Dubin L, Becker M, Hotchkiss RS (1967) Venography in the subfertile man with varicocele. J Urol 98:388
6. Chatel A, Bigot JM, Dectot H, Helenon Ch (1978) Anatomie radiologique des veines spermatiques. J Chir (Paris) 115:443
7. Chatel A, Bigot JM, Barret F, Helenon Ch (1979) Veines spermatiques, voies de suppleance. J Radiol 60:221
8. Comhaire F, Kunnen M (1976) Selective retrograde venography of the internal spermatic vein: A conclusive approach to the diagnosis of varicocele. Andrologia 8:11
9. Dubin L, Amelar RD (1975) Varicocelectomy as therapy in male infertility: A study of 504 cases. Fertil Steril 26:217
10. Etriby A, Ibrahim A, Mahmoud KZ, Elhagaar S (1975) Subfertility and varicocele I. Venogram demonstration of anastomosis sites in subfertile men. Fertil Steril 26:1013
11. Gösfay S (1959) Untersuchungen der Vena spermatica interna durch retrograde Phlebographie bei Kranken mit Varicocele. Z Urol 2:105
12. Hill JT, Green NA (1977) Varicocele: a review of radiological and anatomical features in relation to surgical treatment. Br J Surg 64:747–752
13. Hochgesand J (1970) Über den Verlauf und die Häufigkeit der retroaortären linken Nierenvene bei menschlichen Feten. Z Anat Entwicklungsgesch 130:207
14. Janson R, Weißbach L (1978) Zur Phlebographie der Vena testicularis bei Varicocelenpersistenz bzw. -rezidiv. ROEFO 129:485
15. Knöner M, Dathe G, Palm V (1973) Verbesserung der Ergebnisse der Varicocelenoperation durch präoperative Serienphlebographien. Verh Dtsch Ges Urol 25:335

16. Lindholmer C, Thulin L, Eliasson R (1975) Semen characteristics before and after ligation of the left internal spermatic veins in men with varicocele. Scand J Urol Nephrol 9:177
17. Ludvik W (1970) Varikocele und Fertilität. Aktuel Urol 3:184
18. Mauss J, Schach H, Scheidt J (1974) Andrologische Untersuchungen bei subfertilen Männern vor und nach Varikocelenoperation. Hautarzt 25:394
19. Oehlmann U, Langkopf B, Richter A, Freitag J (1976) Intravasale Nierenvenendruckmessung und selektive renale Phlebographie bei Patienten mit idiopathischer Varikocele. Z Urol 69:643
20. Ortmann R (1968) Über Bedeutung, Häufigkeit und Variationsbild der linken retro-aortären Nierenvene. Z Anat Entwicklungsgesch 127:346
21. Riedl P (1979) Selektive Phlebographie und Katheterthrombosierung der Vena testicularis bei primärer Varikocele. Wr Klin [Suppl] 91:99
22. Riedl P. Retroaortale Nierenvenen – eine mögliche Ursache der linksseitigen Varicocele. ROEFO 133:477
23. Riedl P, Lunglmayr G, Stackl W. A new method of transfemoral testicular vein obliteration for Varicocele using a ballon catheter. Radiology 139:323
24. Rost A, Richter-Reichhelm M, Kaden R, Pust R (1975) Die Varicocele als Ursache von Fertilitätsstörungen. Urologe [A] 14:282
25. Thelen M, Weisbach L, Franken Th (1979) Die Behandlung der idiopathischen Varicocele durch transfemorale Spiralokklusion der Vena testicularis sinistra. ROEFO 131:24
26. Weber J (1978) Phlebographie und Venendruckmessung im Abdomen und Becken. Witzstrock, Baden-Baden Köln New York
27. Zeitler E, Jecht E, Herzinger R, Richter EJ, Seyferth W, Grosse-Vorholt R (1979) Technik und Ergebnisse der Spermatica-Phlebographie bei 136 Männern mit primärer Sterilität. ROEFO 131:179

Phlebography of the Right Spermatic Vein in Varicoceles

J. M. BIGOT, F. BARRET, and C. HELENON

The clinical predominance of varicoceles on the left side first induced radiologists to perform phlebographic examinations of the left spermatic vein. This procedure can easily be performed since the orifice of the left spermatic vein is nearly always on the lower side of the renal vein.

Catheterization of the spermatic vein on the right side is much more difficult because height and location of its opening into the inferior caval vein cary. To date, only a few publications on this procedure are available.

Technique

One should look for the right spermatic vein on the right anterolateral or the anterior side of the inferior caval vein at the height of the transverse process of the second vertebral body by the Seldinger technique using preshaped catheters (in the Tenon Hospital, Biotrol). Contrast material is injected under a Valsalva maneuver into the inferior caval vein and in this way the orifice of the spermatic vein can often be localized. Moreover, this vein frequently anastomoses with the lumbar venous system so that the opacification can also be performed by catheterization of the lumbar collaterals. If these procedures fail, one can inject contrast material into the right renal vein while the patient is in an inclined position and then look here for an opening of the spermatic vein.

At this point some target pictures should be made of the lumbar section to study the anatomic variations. Subsequently, two or at maximum three pictures should be made of the scrotal region with the patient supine in the position and under the Valsalva maneuver. If there is no reflux to the pampiniform plexus, the injection should be made with the patient is in an upright position, and a picture of the scrotum should be taken when the injection is finished.

We use a 32% solution of contrast material. The average dose is 1.5–1.8 ml, and the total dosage is 20–25 ml depending on the size of the spermatic vein.

An effective Valsalva maneuver is necessary to obtain an excellent retrograde flow to the pampiniform plexus. The patient must not be in an upright position when the examination is carried out with a classic angiographic apparatus.

Results

To date, we have carried out 230 phlebographies of the right spermatic vein. At the beginning, the success rate was low but increased to 92% in the last 150 patients with a success rate of 98%–99% on the left side.

Thanks to the increasing experience of the radiologists, knowledge of the numerous anatomic variations, and the localization by Valsalva maneuver, visualization of the right spermatic vein has become a relatively easy procedure.

Anatomic Situation of the Right Spermatic Vein in the Radiogram

Height and location of the orifice of the right spermatic vein vary. In 95% of cases the right spermatic vein opens into the inferior caval vein, and in 5% of cases into the right renal vein.

When entering the inferior caval vein, the orifice is on the right anterior side in 88% of cases and on the left anterior side in 7%. The height of the orifice of the spermatic vein varies as follows:

1. In 46% of cases at the height of the transverse process of the vertebra L 2.
2. In 29% of cases at the height of the intervertebral space L 1–L 2 or the transverse process of L 1.
3. In 25% of cases at the height of the intervertebral space L 2–L 3 or the transverse process of L 3.

Therefore, one must first look for the spermatic vein at the height of the transverse process of L 2 on the right side of the inferior caval vein.

The spermatic vein can also end in two branches into the inferior caval vein (in 6.6%) (Fig. 1 b) or into the inferior caval vein and into the right renal vein (in 16.7%).

The spermatic vein usually appears as a single cord in the lumbar section (Fig. 1). A valve can be found in the orifice of this cord or some centimeters before it (Fig. 1 a). Normally, the valves are in the spermatic vein at the height of the pelvic and upper inguinal section.

The lumen size of the right spermatic vein is not essentially conditioned by the existence of a varicocele. Decisive for the lumen, however, is the size of the intestinal venous trunk (anastomoses with the right intestinal venous system) which meets it on its right side at the height of the iliac crest. At voluminous intestinal venous trunk the spermatic vein, too, is voluminous.

Anastomoses of the right spermatic vein occur in the following ways:

a) The right spermatic vein frequently anastomoses with the right renal vein, for we found that only in 5% of the cases did the spermatic vein open into the renal vein, and that beside the main orifice into the caval vein in 16.7%, another parallel normal calibrated trunk opened into the renal vein. In about 5% of the cases one can find indirect anastomoses between the lumbar section of the right spermatic vein and the renal vein. However, they are less frequent than on the left side (15%).

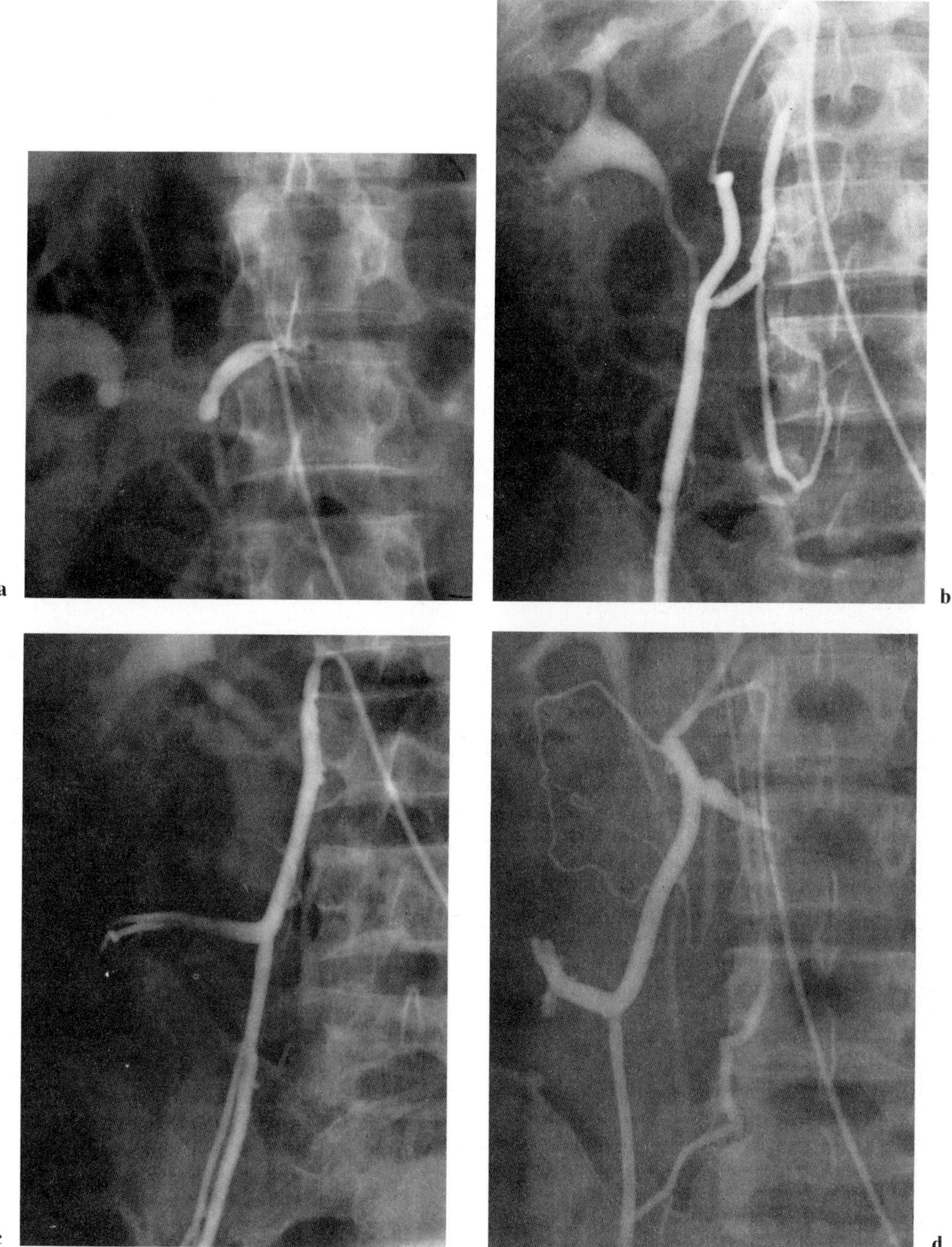

Fig. 1 a–d. Normal right spermatic vein in the lumbar section. (Four different patients)

b) Anastomoses with the external venous system are frequent, between 15% and 18%, but less frequent than on the left side.

c) Anastomoses with intercostal veins are less frequent on the right (4.6%) than on the left side (15.2%). Often, they are joined to the extrarenal venous system as well as to the lumbar and intercostal veins.

d) Anastomoses with the lumbar system and the venous network of the perivertebral system are less frequent on the right (7.7%) than on the left side (40.8%). They are thin-calibrated internal anastomoses which often are arranged stepwise to the ascendent lumbar and perivertebral venous system (Fig. 1 B).

e) Direct anastomoses with the inferior caval vein are thin collaterals, more frequent on the right (7.8%) than on the left side (1.6%). This can be explained by the specific location of the spermatic vein (Fig. 1 D).

f) Anastomoses with the periureteral veins are less frequent on the right (7.8%) than on the left side (19.2%), but we have not yet found a higher rate of periureteral venous dilatations in patients with bilharziasis.

g) Anastomoses among the different sections of the spermatic vein are less frequent on the right (25%) than on the left side (45%). They are thin collaterals arranged

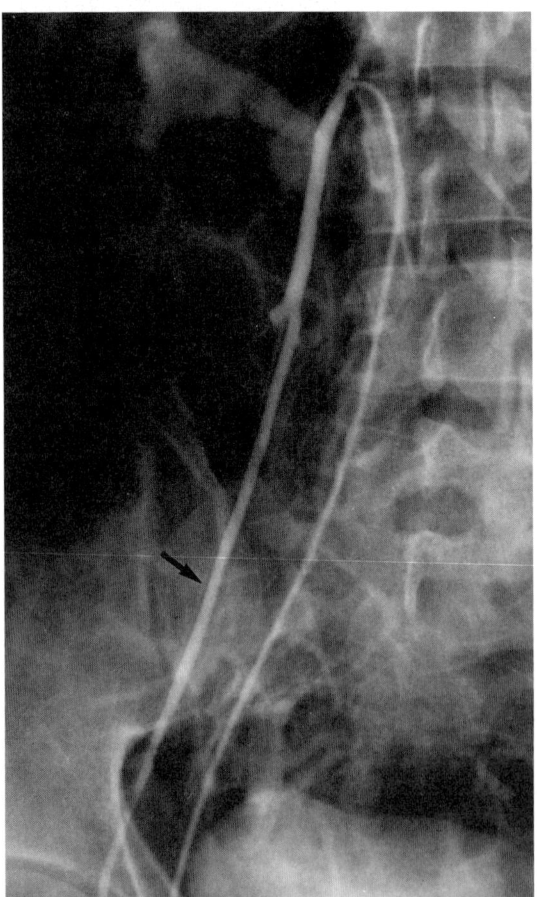

Fig. 2. Anatomic variation. A collateral is seen which begins in the superior lumbar section and which only follows the normal course of the spermatic vein near the inferior orifice of the inguinal channel. This collateral can be the cause of persistency after ligature

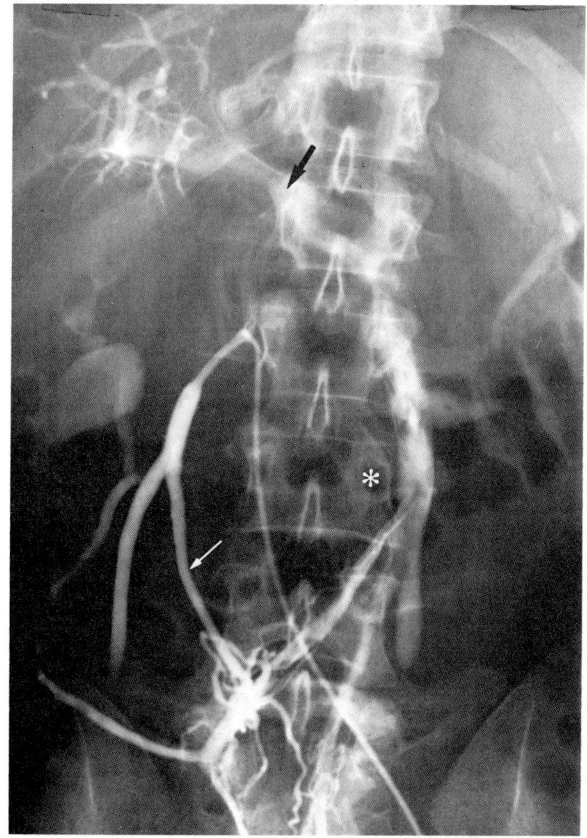

Fig. 3. Anastomosis of the spermatic vein with the superior mesenteric vein: ↗, anastomosis; *, right mesenteric vein; ↙, portal venous trunk

stepwise, both in the lumbar section and in the sections below. Overlooked collaterals in the pelvic section usually are the cause of persistency. The hydrostatic pressure later dilates these overlooked collaterals which then again supply the varicocele (Fig. 2).

h) Often, we can find anastomoses between the right spermatic vein and the portal veins, i.e., with the superior mesenteric vein via the trunk of the intestinal vein (frequency rate 39.5%), usually located on the right border of the right spermatic vein, level with the iliac crest or slightly above it (Fig. 3). Normally, this trunk has a valve 1 or 2 cm before its opening into the spermatic vein (Fig. 1 C and D). Anastomoses with the mesenteric system, however, can only be visualized at the missing valve. The frequency of this anastomosis with the spermatic vein on level with the peritoneal suspension of the colon on the right side is the explanation for the surprising branch-off we found at portal hypertension. In the latter case, contrast material injected into the celiac trunk first produces an opacification against the normal blood stream of the superior mesenteric vein and then a drainage via the right testicular system to the inferior caval vein. We realized this direct opacification of the superior mesenteric vein about 20 times; thus it follows that the intestinal venous trunk is an anastomosis between the portal venous system and that of the spermatic vein. In some cases the anastomosis of the intestinal vein communicates with the parietal veins.

Except for the communications to the inferior caval vein, the anastomoses of the spermatic vein are less frequent on the right side than on the left. The frequency of anastomoses with the portal system is nearly identical on both sides.

Frequency and Definition of the Right-Sided Varicocele

In France, the frequency of varicocele is 3%–10%, at an average rate of 7%. In cases of male infertility, however, this rate is even higher and fluctuates between 9% and 19%, at an average rate of 14%.

The last 100 varicoceles we have shown by phlebography are as follows: bilateral varicoceles, 53; left unilateral varicoceles, 27; and right unilateral varicoceles, 20.

This means that in 73% of the cases we found a varicocele on the right side and in 80% on the left. The frequent occurrence of a unilateral varicocele on the right side (20%) seems interesting for such a value is not mentioned in the available literature.

The definition of a varicocele on the right side is problematic. The varicocele can be diagnosed clinically, thermographically, and radiologically. If the results of these three procedures coincide, no problem arises. If either the clinical or the thermographic method delivers a positive result, the radiologic findings will not be doubted either. But there are also cases of infraclinical varicoceles in which thermographic proof fails because of the size of the left varicocele, and in which phlebography of the spermatic vein reveals a retrograde flow to the pampiniform plexus with varicouse dilatations in this section.

In only a relatively few cases (15%–20%) did we succeed in opacifying the spermatic vein upon injection of contrast material into the inferior caval vein, under the Valsalva maneuver and with the patient in the supine position. In most cases we had to catheterize the vein to obtain retrograde filling to the pampiniform plexus. A varicocele can be ruled out, if valves are visualized which also close well when the patient is in an upright position and which hinder the retrograde flow beyond or beneath the level of the iliac crest. On the other hand, we also had patients in whom we noted not only a retrograde flow to the pampiniform plexus but also a stasis on this level and visualization of more or less voluminous varicoceles after catheterization of the right caval vein. If, however, an opacification in the supine position fails, a varicocele can be excluded on the right side in a patient in an upright and physiologic position.

Upon injection of contrast material into the renal vein, a retrograde flow into the spermatic vein cannot always be noted on the left side. Again and again we had patients in whom catheterization manifested valves in the spermatic vein, and also patients without valves but with varicoceles. These results are not doubted for the left side. However, we presume that on the right side these results are disregarded since a phlebography is seldom performed in these cases.

Varicoceles on the right side are of varying sizes: 25% small, 40% medium, and 35% large (Fig. 4).

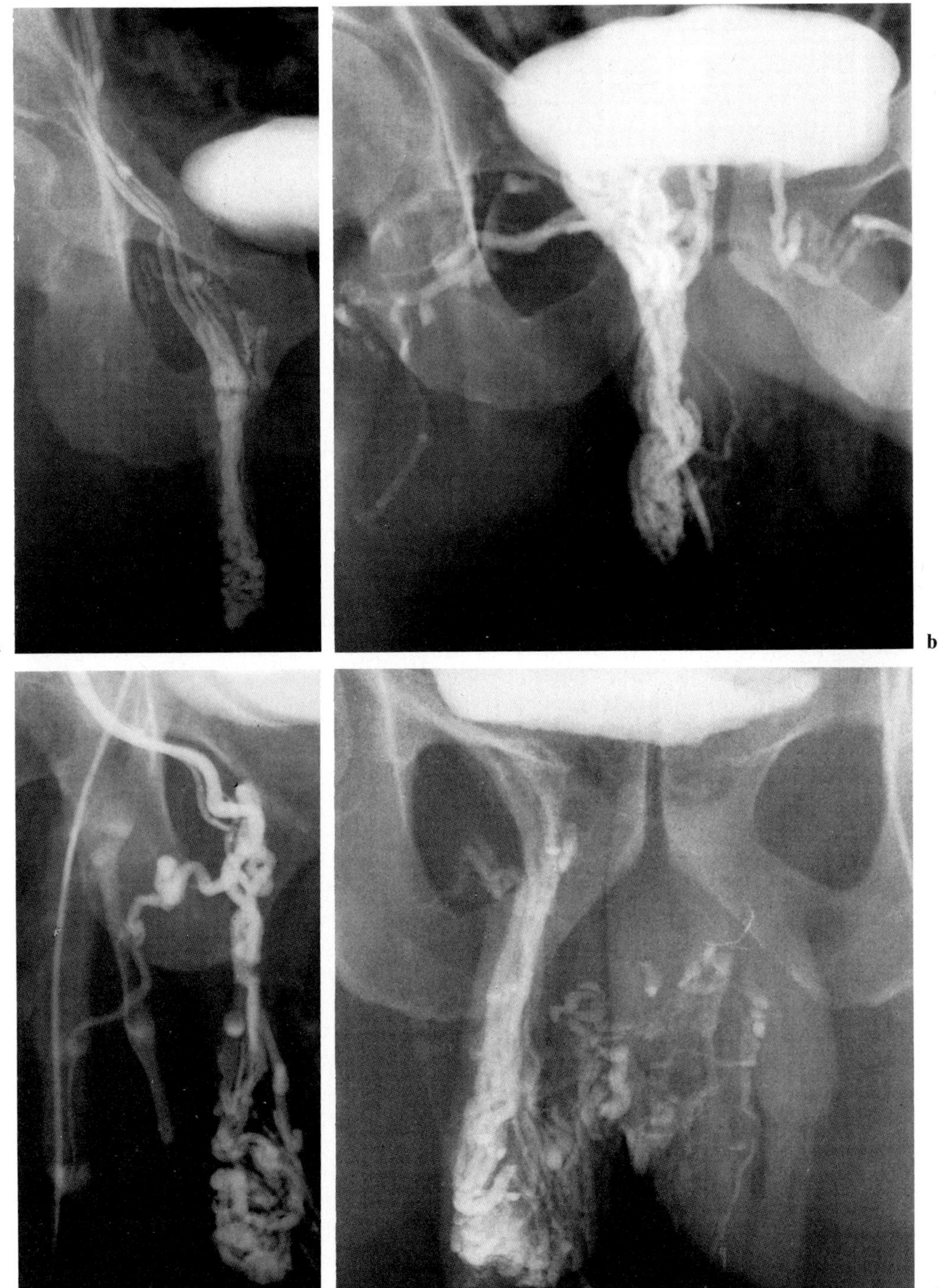

Fig. 4a–d. Different sizes of the varicoceles on the right side. **a** small; **b** medium, drainage into the external pudendal vein; **c** large, drainage into the right femoral vein; and **d** large, with voluminous dilatations at the height of the inguinal channel

Often one can find a persistent varicocele on the left side in patients after an Ivanissevich operation. However, more often an overlooked varicocele on the right side is the reason for a non-improvement of the clinical and thermographic result following surgery.

Only twice in our practice did we find a varicocele on the right side which drained into a left varicocele via a transscrotal path. This is an anatomically unusual fact. In two cases we found a varicocele on the left side which drained into a right varicocele via the same transscrotal path.

The drainage of the right varicocele takes place in the same way as on the left side, i.e., to the external pudendal veins, to the deferential veins, to the external iliac veins, and to the hypogastric veins. If, upon injection of contrast material into the renal or inferior caval vein while the patient is in a supine position, a retrograde flow to the spermatic vein on the right side can be noted, this gives hints with regard to the patency of the spermatic vein. The patency or nonpatency of the trunk does not prove the existence or nonexistence of a varicocele on the right side.

There are patent veins which, because of a voluminous intestinal trunk, have a rather large lumen with valves at the height of the pelvis that prevent retrograde flow to the pampiniform plexus. On the other hand, there are right spermatic veins which, in spite of contrast material injection into the inferior caval vein and under Valsalva maneuver, cannot be visualized. These veins, after selective catheterization, appear completely free of valves and a relatively large varicocele can be demonstrated radiologically. Thus, in our opinion, a varicocele on the right side can be defined as a retrograde flow of contrast material to the pampiniform plexus with varicose dilatations in this section.

Etiology

The cause of a varicocele might be the upright position with retrograde flow or a stasis in the spermatic vein. Naturally, valve insufficiency favors this development.

A varicocele on the left side also may be the sign of a thrombosis in the left renal vein, and, if a varicocele only recently has developed, one should look for a renal tumor.

In some cases with thromboses in the femoral and in the iliac vein we noted opacification of the pampiniform plexus from the external pudendal vein, and then a drainage via the spermatic vein in an orthograde ascending peripheral venous flow. This is an anastomosis from caval vein to caval vein caused by a voluminous thrombosis.

We have not yet been able to visualize a postoperatively persistent varicocele on contrast material injection into the external iliac vein with the patient in an upright position. In all our cases with persistency, we found a contrast material accumulation below the ligature caused by thin-calibrated collaterals which were overlooked in the first operation.

Indication of Phlebography

Phlebography of the spermatic vein in cases of male infertility is indicated when clinical and thermographic examinations have been made in addition to two spermiograms after hormone determination (testosterone, estradiol, FSH, LH, prolactin).

When compared to the radiological results, clinical examinations reveal negative findings in 36% of the cases on the left side and in 74% on the right side. This difference demonstrates that, on the one hand, the right-sided varicocele remained undiscovered clinically or was even misinterpreted, e.g., as hydrocele and that, on the other hand, the right-sided varicocele is often smaller than on the left side.

About 14% of the left-sided varicoceles remained undiscovered when thermography was used, against 48% on the right side. The reason is that bilateral varicoceles are often dominated by the left-sided varicocele, and the right-sided varicocele therefore remains undiscovered. In total, 21% of the subclinical varicoceles are not discovered by thermography and can only be visualized with a bilateral phlebography of the spermatic vein. Thermography of bilateral varicoceles neither shows whether one of them is supplied from the contralateral clarify side. This seldom occurs but one must know the correct side when an operation is indicated.

Spermatological Results

It was rather difficult to obtain the results of the 250 operations with the Ivanissevich technique, for the French do not like to give information about themselves. Nevertheless, spermiograms made in numerous patients 3–6 months later showed a significant improvement in 50%–60%. A study is now being carried out to register the number of pregnancies.

Conclusion

The frequency of right-sided varicocele can be shown by phlebography of the spermatic vein. This frequency could not be clinically diagnosed and the assessment by means of thermographic and sonographic examinations failed. The effects of the right-sided varicocele on the spermatogenesis on the right side are uncertain, as is the question of whether the factors of stasis and anoxia are decisive or whether the factors of stasis and anoxia are decisive or whether their role is only a secondary one in comparison with the retrograde flow of catecholamines from the renal venous system. In the first case the radiologic examination is indispensible in proving the existence of a varicocele. When there is a missing retrograde flow from the renal system and when this fact is considered decisive, the radiologically proved varicocele might not have an influence on the spermatogenesis.

Phlebography of the right spermatic vein can be performed with nearly the same rate as on the left side. Phlebography is absolutely necessary in cases of lack of improvement of semen quality, for we frequently noted that varicoceles on the right side primary were overlooked.

Technique, Indications, and Results of Transfemoral Phlebography of the Testicular Vein in Persistent Varicocele

R. JANSON and L. WEISSBACH

In the majority of cases, the varicocele operation is a failure because of the persistence of the varicocele, and not because of a real recurrence. In the literature [2, 3, 4, 6], the average percentage of failure for the different operation techniques is about 10%. In our two clinics, therefore, the general indication for transfemoral phlebography of the testicular vein is given only in the case of a persistent varicocele before the reoperation. Preoperative knowledge of the testicular venous drainage routes and the numerous possible venous shunts greatly influences the choice of surgical procedure and helps to diminish the rate of postoperative persistences or recurrences. For this reason we increasingly do transfemoral phlebography in the primary diagnostics.

The *technique of retrograde phlebography* of the testicular vein is described in detail in many publications [2, 5, 6, 7]. It is important that the reflux into the testicular vein is examined by injection into the renal as well as into the testicular vein. In addition, the reflux should be checked with the patient in a standing position and under the conditions of a Valsalva maneuver. We used meglumine iothalamate (Conray 30, Fa. Byk Gulden) at low concentration as contrast medium.

Patient Data and Results

Twenty-six patients with persistent varicoceles were examined by transfemoral phlebography of the testicular vein before the second-look operation. In 16 cases the first surgical intervention was a so-called suprainguinal ligature according to Bernardi. In five cases a so-called intrainguinal ligature according to Ivanissevich was done and one young patient was treated by a so-called subinguinal ligature according to Narrath. Two patients had already been operated on twice without success and one patient had even been operated on three times. In one case the exact kind of operation was unknown.

The most important result of this investigation of the second-look operation was proof of the reflux into one or more branches of the testicular vein in 25 of the 26 cases. In one case an additional scrotal phlebography was necessary; we found a reflux presumably coming from the external spermatic vein via the inferior epigastric vein and the external iliac vein [1, 2]. We also saw the known venous shunts to the renal capsule and renal pelvis veins, to the ureter veins, to the azygos-hemiazygos system and the paravertebral system, to the pelvic and the other retroperitoneal veins. These anatomically preformed collaterals are partially collapsed during the surgical intervention, so that they are easily overlooked. Later they can become hemodynamically effective for the collateral circulation with connections to the distal trunk of the testicular vein. In the majority of cases we could localize the site of the former ligature and resection fairly well.

To summarize retrograde phlebography of the testicular vein is the method of choice for proving the persistent reflux after an unsuccessful operation of a varicocele. It is the only method which shows the pathophysiology of testicular venous drainage and therefore it will be used increasingly for preoperative planning in the surgical treatment of varicoceles.

References

1. Hanley HG, Harrison RG (1962) The nature and treatment of varicocele. Br J Surg 56:64
2. Janson R, Weißbach L (1978) Zur Phlebographie der Vena testicularis bei Varikozelen-persistenz bzw. -rezidiv. ROEFO 129/4:485
3. Klosterhalfen H, Schirren C (1968) Die operative Behandlung der Varicocele. Chir Praxis 12:425
4. Lindholmer C (1975) Semen characteristics before and after ligation of the left internal spermatic veins in men with varicocele. Scand J Urol Nephrol 9:177
5. Riedl P (1979) Selektive Phlebographie und Katheterthrombosierung der Vena testicularis bei primärer Varikozele. Eine angiographisch-anatomische und klinische Studie. Wien Klin Wochenschr [Suppl] 91/9:99
6. Weißbach L, Janson R (1979) Die transfemorale Phlebographie der Vena testicularis vor der Operation des sog. Varikozelen-Rezidivs. In: Reinterventionen an den Urogenitalorganen, Weber W, Jonas D, eds. Thieme Stuttgart, p 280
7. Zeitler E, Jecht E, Herzinter R, Richter E-I, Seyferth W, Grosse-Vorholt R (1979) Technik und Ergebnisse der Spermatica-Phlebographie bei 136 Männern mit primärer Sterilität. ROEFO 131/2:179

B. Other Methods

The Value of Physical Examination for the Diagnosis of Varicocele

E. W. Jecht, R. Herzinger, and E. Zeitler

Varicoceles have been described as a "grape-sized mass" [8], a "palpable scrotal varicosity" [7], or an "abnormal dilatation and coiling of the veins within the *plexus pampiniformis*" [1] of varying degree. There are many more similar characterizations of varicoceles [9], and all are based on an alteration of scrotal veins perceptible by palpation. Whether palpability really is a common feature of varicoceles has been made dubious by the discovery of the nonpalpable "subclinical" varicocele [3].

Since this discovery, retrograde flow down the internal spermatic vein has been – and still is – considered the common denominator for clinical *and* subclinical varicoceles [9]. "Selective retrograde venography of the internal spermatic vein" is the only "conclusive approach to the diagnosis of varicocele" [2].

We have investigated 128 patients for the presence of a reflux in the left internal spermatic vein by percutaneous selective phlebography [10]. These patients had consulted us for treatment of sterility and were all found to produce semen of reduced quality. The rationale for the venography was:

1. To clarify whether or not a subclinical varicocele, i.e., retrograde flow down the internal spermatic vein, was evident in patients without clinical (palpable) varicocele.
2. To verify a reflux in the internal spermatic vein in patients with clinical varicocele.
3. To minimize the rate of postoperative persistent varicoceles (see this symposium) by providing the surgeon with the X-ray plates of the phlebography.

Clinical and radiological results are summarized in Table 1. Of the 54 patients without clinical evidence for a varicocele, 28 were found to demonstrate a reflux in

Table 1. Results of clinical examination for left-sided varicocele and selective phlebography of left internal spermatic vein in 128 patients with reduced semen quality

Clinical examination		Selective phlebography	
	n	Reflux	No Reflux
Varicocele	74	48	26
No varicocele	54	28	26
n	128	76	52

the left internal spermatic vein. Thus, a subclinical varicocele was discovered in 22% of the 128 patients with reduced semen quality. In other words, the palpatory finding was "false negative" in 22% of the 128 patients. While a certain percentage of patients with a subclinical varicocele was to be – and had been – expected, the absence of a reflux in patients with a clinical varicocele came as a surprise. A retrograde flow down the left internal spermatic vein could be verified in only 48 of the 74 patients with a clinical varicocele on the left side. In 20% of the 128 patients in this study, therefore, a clinical varicocele without reflux in the internal spermatic vein was evident.

There are several possible explanations for these "false positive" clinical varicoceles:

1. Eagerness on the part of the examining physician to detect subclinical varicoceles
2. Reflux in the external spermatic vein [4]
3. The presence of a posttraumatic varicocele [5]
4. Nonselective catheterization of the internal spermatic vein due to anatomical anomalies or insufficient technique.

Whatever the explanation, high ligation of the internal spermatic vein would very likely have been done without success in these patients with "false positive" varicocele before the era of phlebography. It is conceivable that similar clinical varicoceles without retrograde flow may have caused failures of improvement in semen quality after high ligation.

In a recent study, absolutely no therapeutic value of high ligation was found in 51 patients with a clinical varicocele and reduced semen quality [6]. It is worth noting that in this study "the evaluation of semen quality from one or more of the crude" [*sic*] "variables such as sperm count or sperm morphology is very often 'a case of beauty being in the eye of the beholder'". However, apparently it was deemed superfluous to consider selective phlebography of the internal spermatic vein and/or thermography and/or the Doppler technique in this study, let alone actually perform these techniques before and after operation. "Manual palpation" alone was the cornerstone of diagnostic endeavour in this study [6]. Lo and behold, the beauty – of false positive varicoceles – lies in the hand of the palpator. Our data conclusively demonstrate that "manual palpation" [6] is insufficient for diagnosis and verification of varicocele, at any rate if "the findings . . . are provocative" [6].

References

1. CIOMS (1976) Krankheiten der Harnorgane und der männlichen Geschlechtsorgane. CIOMS-Projekt, Band 5, Heidelberg
2. Comhaire F, Kunnen M (1976) Selective retrograde venography of the internal spermatic vein: A conclusive approach to the diagnosis of varicocele. Andrologia 8:11
3. Comhaire F, Monteyne R, Kunnen M (1976) The value of scrotal thermography as compared with selective retrograde venography of the internal spermatic vein for the diagnosis of "subclinical" varicocele. Fertil Steril 27:694
4. Hill JT, Green NA (1977) Varicocele: A review of radiological and anatomical features in relation to surgical treatment. Br J Surg 64:747
5. Hornstein OP (1973) Kreislaufstörungen im Hoden-Nebenhodensystem und ihre Bedeutung für die männliche Fertilität. Andrologia 5:119

6. Nilsson S, Edvinsson A, Nilsson B (1979) Improvement of semen and pregnancy rate after ligation and division of the internal spermatic vein: Fact or fiction? Br J Urol 51:591
7. Steeno O, Knops J, Declerck L, Adimoelja A, Van De Voorde H (1976) Prevention of fertility disorders by detection and treatment of varicocele at school and college age. Andrologia 8:47
8. Uehling DT (1968) Fertility in men with varicocele. Int J Fertil 13:58
9. Verstoppen GR, Steeno OP (1977) Varicocele and the pathogenesis of the associated subfertility – a review of the various theories. I: Varicocelogenesis. Andrologia 9:133
10. Zeitler E, Jecht E, Herzinger R, Richter E-I, Seyferth W, Grosse-Vorholt R (1979) Technik und Ergebnisse der Spermatica-Phlebographie bei 136 Männern mit primärer Sterilität. ROEFO 131:179

Contact Thermography in the Diagnosis of Varicocele

P. RIEDL and W. STACKL

The value of infrared and contact thermography in the diagnosis of varicoceles is repeatedly stressed [3, 4, 8]. While the technique is reported to be particularly useful for demonstrating so-called subclinical varicoceles, it has equally been employed for monitoring the success of transfemoral testicular vein obliteration [6, 7].

In this contribution we will review the diagnostic thermographies performed on 144 patients and the 57 cases monitored after testicular vein obliteration.

Material and Method

A total of 144 patients, aged between 13 and 48 years, who underwent treatment for varicocele at the University of Vienna Medical School were examined. Thermograms were compared with palpatory findings, spermiograms, and, in 134 cases, with selective testicular vein phlebograms.

For examinations, an ELC contact thermograph (CAWO Comp.) with integrated slide camera was used. Thermograph plates were calibrated for 31 °C, 32 °C, and 33 °C, and the difference to the normal contralateral side was recorded. Temperatures were equalized with a hand blower. In the cases treated by transfemoral testicular vein obliteration (n = 57), thermography was done 2 days, 1 week, and 1, 3, 6, and 12 months after treatment for monitoring the course of the condition.

Positive findings were rated in three grades:

Grade I (↑):	Minor marginal rise of temperature over a small part of the scrotum (usually laterocranial)
Grade II (↑↑):	Temperature rise over approximately half of the scrotum
Grade III (↑↑↑):	Massive rise of temperature over the entire scrotum on the disease side.

Clinically, varicoceles were allocated to three size groups [2]; so-called subclinical varicoceles (doubtful palpatory findings on Valsava maneuver and abnormal spermiogram) constituted a separate fourth group [1].

Grade I (+):	Small varicoceles escaping inspection: on palpation the diameter of the venous package is less than 1 cm
Grade II (++):	Varicoceles that may be missed on simple inspection; diameter 1 to 2 cm
Grade III (+++):	Varicoceles visible from a distance; diameter more than 2 cm.

Results

Table 1 compares diagnostic contact thermograms with clinical varicocele size and phlebograms. Large varicoceles invariably gave positive findings on thermography. In a single case the varicocele mechanism was not demonstrable on selective retrograde phlebography. An antegrade (scrotal) venogram was not obtainable because the patient did not come back as scheduled. Medium-sized and small varicoceles failed to show on the thermograms in 14 cases. However, a varicocele mechanism was demonstrable on phlebography in 12 cases. Results obtained in the group classified as subclinical varicoceles are shown in Table 2. A varicocele mechanism was not demonstrable in five of the cases with abnormal thermograms. It was, however, visualized in one patient with a normal thermogram.

Table 3 compares contact thermography with clinical palpation after transfemoral obliteration. The figures listed relate to the number of examinations for each sclerosing treatment rather than to the number of patients. Of the 57 patients, seven underwent treatment twice and one bilaterally. After treatment in patients without palpatory evidence of a varicocele, the first posttreatment thermography

Table 1. Palpatory findings, contact thermography, and phlebography in 144 patients with varicocele

N	%	Palpation	Contact thermography				Normal	Phlebography		Not done
			Abnormal					Varicocele mechanism		
			$\uparrow$	$\uparrow\uparrow$	$\uparrow\uparrow\uparrow$	total		Present	Absent	
47	32.6	+ + +	9	8	30	47	–	45	1	1
27	18.8	+ +	8	14	–	22	5	27	–	–
41	28.5	+	24	8	–	32	9	36	2	3
29	20.1		10	1	–	11	18	10	13	6
144	100.0		51	31	30	112	32	118	16	10

Table 2. Contact thermography and phlebography in 29 patients with subclinical varicocele

Thermography	n	Phlebography		Not done
		Varicocele mechanism		
		Present	Absent	
Positive	11	5	5	1
Negative	18	1	12	5
	29			

Table 3. Contact thermography and palpation before. 1 week, 3 months, and 6 to 12 months after transfemoral testicular vein obliteration ($n=65$)

n	%	Clinical findings after obliteration	Contact thermography																			
			Pretreatment					1 day – 1 week					3 months					6 – 12 months				
			↓		↑	↑↑	↑↑↑	↓		↑	↑↑	↑↑↑	↓		↑	↑↑	↑↑↑	↓		↑	↑↑	↑↑↑
52	80.0	Varicocele not palpable	2	5	22	16	7	9	34	9	–	–	3	35	1	–	–	5	14	–	–	–
9	13.8	Varicocele smaller	–	1	–	3	5	1	–	6	2	–	–	–	3	4	–	–	–	–	–	–
4	6.2	Varicocele unchanged	–	–	1	1	2	–	–	1	1	2	–	–	1	1	2	–	–	–	–	–
65	100.0																					

showed a slightly reduced temperature over the left scrotum in nine cases, while another nine still had slightly elevated temperatures on the left. (These thermographies were mostly obtained on the first or second posttreatment days.) Within 3 months the temperature differences disappeared in almost all cases.

Except in one case, all patients with complete or partial varicocele persistence had consistently elevated posttreatment temperatures on the diseased side.

Discussion

As shown in Tables 1 and 2, contact thermography gave incorrect results in 18 (13.4%) of the phlebographically verified cases. The failure rate increases to 20.5% if only medium-sized and small as well as subclinical varicoceles are considered and large (grade III) varicoceles are excluded. In the latter, thermography and phlebography were invariably found to agree. The failure to demonstrate a varicocele mechanism in a grade III varicocele on selective retrograde phlebography, in spite of clearly abnormal contact thermography and clinical examination in one of our cases, appears to be due to filling of the dilated veins from other sources (external spermatic vein and/or deferential vein).

What factors might possibly account for the failure rate of the technique in small and subclinical varicoceles? One factor could well be inherent in the technique itself. Infrared thermography, which gives more accurate temperature measurements, appears to be superior to contact thermography [8]. Cooling of the skin with a hand blower might constitute another factor. As examinations were carried out in the mammography unit, it was impossible to allow for a 10-min acclimatization of the patients to the ambient room temperature, as proposed by Gasser et al. [3]. In addition, the Valsalva maneuver was omitted.

As Comhaire et al., Gasser et al., and Kormano et al. equally reported variable failure rates and those published by Lewis and Harrison are comparable to ours, it is quite possible that the technique is consistently associated with a failure rate of about 10%–20% in subclinical and small varicoceles.

Failures included both normal thermographies in cases with angiographically verified reflux (grade I and grade II varicoceles) and slightly abnormal thermograms in cases without reflux on angiography (subclinical varicoceles).

For monitoring the success of sclerosing treatment, thermography proved to give excellent results. In cases with complete clinical disappearance of the varicocele the temperature on the diseased side was found either to drop or continue to be elevated for some days. However, these temperature differences tend to disappear within some months. Persisting or relapsing varicoceles were found to be truthfully reflected by the temperature recordings. One possible explanation for the varying reliability of diagnostic versus posttreatment thermographies might be that, as the previous trace is available for comparison with the posttreatment thermograms, even minor differences in the findings obtained can be better interpreted.

Summary

Contact thermography was carried out for diagnostic purposes in 144 cases with suspected varicocele (134 of them equally undergoing angiography for verification) and in 57 patients for monitoring the outcome of transfemoral testicular vein obliteration. In grade III varicocele, diagnostic thermography was found to produce correct positive results throughout. In 12 of 68 patients with medium-sized or small varicoceles demonstrable on angiography, thermography was noncontributory. Five patients with subclinical varicoceles had abnormal thermography, but a varicocele mechanism was not visualized on angiography. If employed for monitoring the success of testicular vein obliteration, thermography consistently produced useful results.

References

1. Comhaire F, Monteyne R, Kunnen M (1976) The value of scrotal thermography as compared with selective retrograde venography of the internal spermatic vein for diagnosis of "subclinical" varicocele. Fertil Steril 27:694
2. Dubin L, Amelar RD (1970) Varicocele size and results of varicocelectomy in selected men with varicocele. Fertil Steril 21:606
3. Gasser G, Strassl R, Pokieser H (1973) Thermogramm des Hodens und Spermiogramm. Andrologia 5:127
4. Kormano M, Kahanpää K, Svinhufvud U, Täthi E (1970) Thermography of varicocele. Fertil Steril 21:558
5. Lewis RW, Harrison RM (1979) Contact scrotal thermography: application to problems of infertility. J Urol 122:40
6. Riedl P (1979) Selektive Phlebographie und Katheterthrombosierung der Vena testicularis bei primärer Varikocele. Wien Klin Wochenschr [Suppl] 91:99
7. Riedl P, Lunglmayr G, Stackl W. A new method of transfemoral testicular vein obliteration for varicocele using a balloon-catheter. Radiology 139:323
8. Zorgniotti AW, Toth AJ (1979) Infrared thermometry for testicular temperature determinations. Fertil Steril 32:347

The Doppler Technique for the Diagnosis of Varicocele

C. MEISEL

The varicocele represents a minor and additional finding in the clientele of my dermatology practice. However, during the first physical examination of dermatologic patients, I find a varicocele in about 15% of all men. Patients referred by an infertility service usually are very cooperative due to the desire to have children; in contrast, patients in the dermatologic practice very often do not care much for problems of fertility and are thus unwilling to undergo further investigations. Therefore, the technique for further investigation of the varicocele should not be time consuming or invasive.

The Doppler technique has become an accepted non-invasive method for the study of reflux in the veins of the legs. It appeared, therefore, worthwhile to study the venous reflux in the spermatic cords of patients with varicoceles.

Theoretically, the following findings can be expected:

1. If a sufficient valve is located superior to the entrance of the spermatic vein into the abdomen, the volume of blood pushed down during the Valsalva maneuver will be small; therefore, only a short reflux is to be expected.
2. If, however, the valve close to the ostium of the internal spermatic vein is sufficient, while all other valves are insufficient or absent, a relatively large volume of blood can be pushed down during the Valsalva maneuver, causing a clear but decreasing regurgitant flow.
3. If all valves in the spermatic vein are insufficient or absent, the blood will continuously flow down during the Valsalva maneuver, causing a strong and continuous regurgitant flow. With normalization of intraabdominal pressure following, the intrascrotal part of the varicocele will be emptied, causing a short antegrade flow.

When using the "Doppler-Sonde"[1], the left hand of the examiner grips the pampiniform plexus, the ring finger accelerating the blood flow with pumping motions, while the right hand keeps the Doppler-Sonde in close contact with the funiculus spermaticus at the entrance into the inguinal canal. After some changes of the location of the Doppler-Sonde, the spot will be found where the flow is best heard. The patient is asked to perform a Valsalva maneuver and the regurgitant flow is recorded.

---

1 Kranzbühler, Modell 280.

The results collected by the Doppler technique, as well as by palpation, semen analysis, and spermatica phlebography, are divided into three classes to allow a somewhat crude correlation.

The flow, recorded with the "Doppler-Sonde", was subdivided into three groups:

1. Pathologic: a strong flow
2. Subnormal: a moderate flow
3. Normal: no or very little flow.

The findings of the clinical examination were classified as follows:
1. Pathologic: grade II and III, according to Steeno et al. [5]
2. Subnormal: grade I [5]
3. Normal: no varicocele palpable.

The values of the sperm count were grouped as follows:
1. Pathologic: less than 15 mill/ml
2. Subnormal: 15–30 mill/ml
3. Normal: more than 30 mill/ml.

Classes for motility:
1. Pathologic: quantitative, less than 30%; qualitative, less than 10%
2. Subnormal: quantitative, 30%–50%; qualitative, 10%–20%
3. Normal: quantitative, 50%; qualitative, 20%.

Classes for morphology:
1. Pathologic: less than 40% normal forms and/or more than 5% spermiogenetic cells
2. Subnormal: 40%–60% normal forms and/or 2%–5% spermiogenetic cells
3. Normal: more than 60% normal forms and less than 2% spermiogenetic cells.

Morphological deformations considered typical for the varicocele [4] were subdivided in a special class. An increase of elongated heads of more than 25% and/or of multinucleated spermatids of more than 5% were considered pathologic (subnormal: 15% and 2%, respectively).

The phlebography of the internal spermatic vein was performed in the radiologic department of the Nürnberg General Hospital. Results were classified as pathologic in cases of insufficiency grade 2 and 3, as subnormal in cases of insufficiency grade 1, and as normal when all valves were sufficient.

When comparing the results of all patients with pathologic Doppler findings, a consistent correspondence was seen in most patients (particularly for morphological seminal parameters).

In the patients with subnormal Doppler results, there was good agreement with clinical and radiologic results while the seminal parameters were almost normal. The number of patients with normal Doppler findings is too small for a conclusive interpretation.

The relationship between the different findings is shown more clearly in the following correlation squares (Figs. 1–3).

When comparing the Doppler findings with the clinical severity of varicoceles, the values are found mostly in the middle squares. It is noteworthy that a normal Doppler result is combined with a clinically large varicocele more often than vice

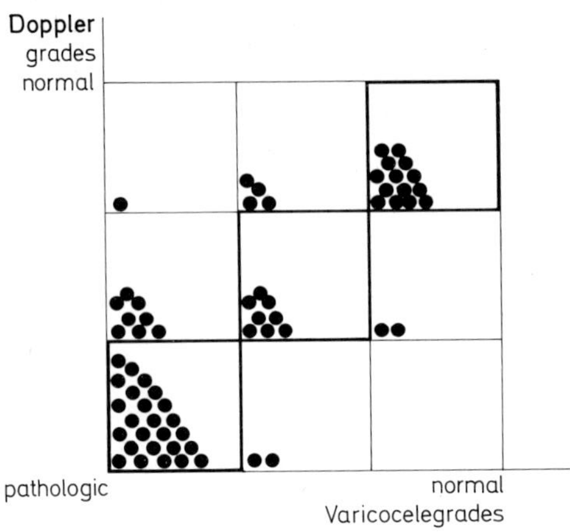

Fig. 1. Doppler findings and clinical grades of varicocele (n = 64)

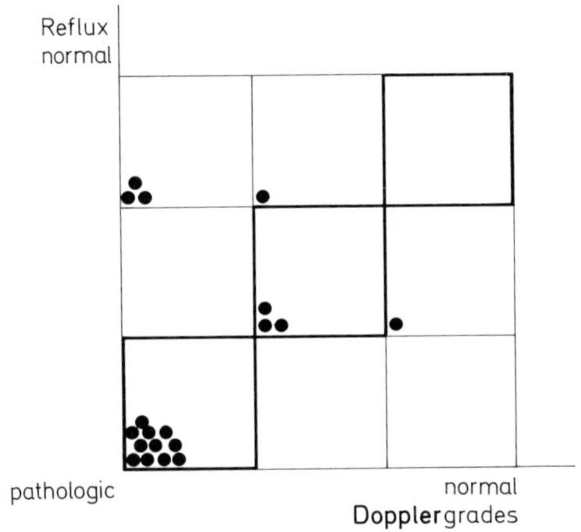

Fig. 2. Doppler findings and results of phlebography (n = 19)

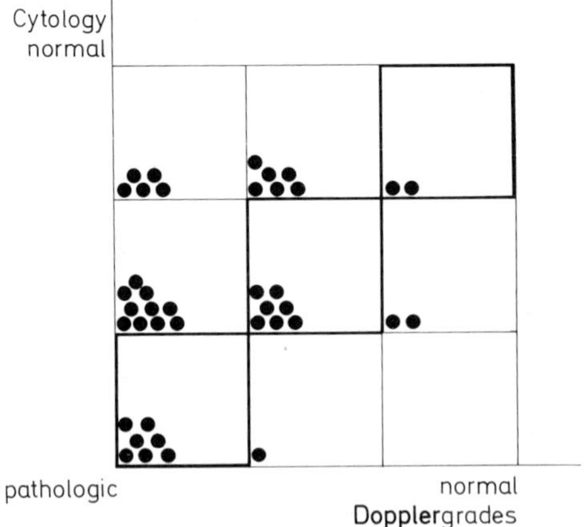

Fig. 3. Doppler findings and seminal cytology (n = 40)

versa (Fig. 1). A similar situation is seen for the radiologic phlebography of the spermatic vein (due to lack of motivation, the number of patients here is much smaller): The pathologic findings of both the Doppler technique and phlebography correspond to a high degree – there are only three patients with a pathologic Doppler finding and a normal phlebography. Patients with normal Doppler results were not sent to the radiologist (Fig. 2).

The comparison of Doppler findings and seminal parameters characteristic for varicocele shows complete coincidence of normal results; however, there are quite a few patients with a pathologic Doppler result and – as yet? – normal seminal parameters (Fig. 3).

Discussion

Greenberg et al. [2] compared the results of clinical examination, semen analysis, and Doppler in 46 patients. They found a good correspondence in the case of large varicoceles but only a slight correspondence in the case of moderate varicoceles. Our results tend to confirm the findings of Greenberg et al. [2]. It has been proposed that the alteration of testicular tissue seen in varicocele is due to a reflux of adrenal substances into the testicular venal system [1, 3]. If this assumption is true – although it does not appear very likely for hemodynamic reasons – an insufficiency of the valves at the ostium of the spermatic vein into the renal vein is necessary. In this case, the effectiveness of the Doppler technique can be controlled by the phlebography of the internal spermatic vein, the latter being the definite proof for an insufficiency of the valve.

My results tend to confirm the assumption of a high correlation between the Doppler technique and phlebography; however, the number of patients as yet examined with those techniques is too small to draw any definite conclusions.

A high intratesticular venous hypertension, on the other hand, is entirely possible, despite sufficiency of the valves at the mouth of the internal spermatic vein. It is conceivable that this hypertension per se may be an important reason for the testicular damage seen in varicocele; if so, the Doppler technique is the better diagnostic tool for the detection or rejection of a varicocele.

The relatively poor correlation of the Doppler findings to seminal parameters is very likely due to the large variation of semen output and quality, and thus no criterion for the effectiveness of the Doppler method.

Further studies will be necessary to clarify the effectiveness of the Doppler technique for the diagnosis of varicoceles. The Doppler technique definitely fulfills the conditions initially required in that it is not time consuming or invasive.

Wutz [6] has shown that a varicocele is detected by physical examination for the service in 2% of men of military age. When doing the physical examination more carefully with respect to the genital area, however, he found a prevalence of 5% of men with a varicocele [6]. The Doppler technique, therefore, should be used for the detection of varicoceles to prevent damage to the testicular tissue.

References

1. Comhaire F, Vermeulen A (1974) Varicocele sterility: cortisol and catecholamines. Fertil Steril 25:88
2. Greenberg StH, Lipshultz LI, Morganroth I, Wein AJ (1977) The use of the Doppler stethoskope in the evaluation of varicocele. J Urol 117:296
3. Lindholmer C, Thulin L, Eliasson R (1973) Concentrations of cortisol and renin in the internal spermatic vein of men with varicocele. Andrologia 5:21
4. MacLeod J (1965) Seminal cytology in the presence of varicocele. Fertil Steril 16:735
5. Steeno O, Knops J, Declerck L, Adimoelia A, van de Voorde H (1976) Prevention of fertility discorders by detection and treatment of varicocele at school and college age. Andrologia 8:47
6. Wutz J (1977) Über die Häufigkeit von Varicocelen und Hodendystopien 19jähriger Männer. Klinikarzt 6:319

Diagnosis and Differential Diagnosis of Varicocele by Ultrasound

A. Gebauer, G. Antes, and G. Staehler

Ultrasound is used more and more in medicine today [1, 2]. There are also reports about ultrasonography examinations of scrotal masses [3, 4, 5]. Ultrasound, however, plays only a minor role in the diagnosis of varicocele. Clinical and angiographic examination are of greater importance, as has been shown before. This paper discusses whether ultrasound is superfluous in the diagnosis and differential diagnosis of varicocele or whether it is still useful and complementary.

In cooperation with the Department of Urology at the University of Munich, we performed ultrasound examinations of the scrotum in 246 patients between 1976 and January, 1980.

Table 1 shows the indications we have worked out for ultrasound examination, based on our patient material [5]. These indications do not include varicocele. Table 2 shows the reasons for giving ultrasound examinations to 246 patients. We performed the examinations only when the palpatory findings were questionable, i.e., in those cases in which ultrasound had to differentiate between varicocele and other

Table 1. Indications for ultrasound of the scrotum

1. Exclusion of a *testicular tumor* in questionable finding on palpation.
   a) previous operations (for hydrocele or spermatocele, resection of the epididymis)
   b) previous trauma
   c) large hydrocele
2. Exclusion of a solid tumor of the epididymis.
3. Proof of an inguinal hernia with a concomitant disease of the scrotal contents.

Table 2. Reasons for performing ultrasound examinations in 246 patients

Pathological palpatory findings, exclusion of a tumor	84
Clinical suspicion of a tumor	21
Hydrocele on palpation, testicle not palpable	36
Inflammations	39
Search for a tumor (elevated sedimation rate, gynecomastia, lymphnodemetastasis)	33
suspicion of a small spermatocele	15
Small varicocele, other disease	12
Hematoma, result of trauma	6

diseases of the scrotal contents. The presence of a varicocele was doubtful in only 12 of 213 patients. This clearly reveals that the clinical diagnosis of varicocele poses no great problem and for this reason varicocele patients were rarely sent for ultrasonographic examinations.

The differential diagnosis includes spermatoceles, inflammatory or tumorous masses of the epididymis, tumors of the testicles, and sometimes small hydroceles.

We performed the ultrasound examinations with a compound scanner and a 5 mHz transducer (6.5 mm diameter) in the recumbent patient. The recumbent position is chosen deliberately; the venous convolute should be emptied in order to recognize the other structures. If there are any diagnostic doubts, the examination is repeated in an upright position after the veins have refilled.

Examples of our findings are demonstrated in Figures 1–6. The normal sonogram of the scrotum (Fig. 1) shows the homogeneous echo pattern of the parenchyma of the testicle. The epididymis can be delimited only by way of intimation and partially within the area of its head. Normal vessels usually are not seen with this technique. The head of the epididymis can be recognized more clearly in the presence of a small hydrocele. It sits on the top of the testicle in a cap-like fashion.

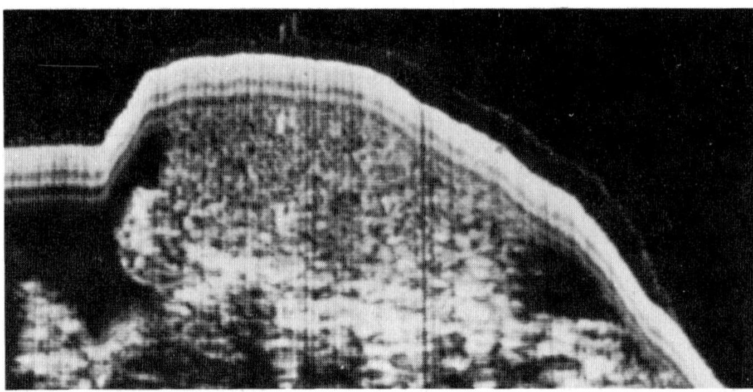

Fig. 1. Varicocele: An echolucent zone with a surrounding echogenic border. The parenchyma of the testicle on the right is unremarkable

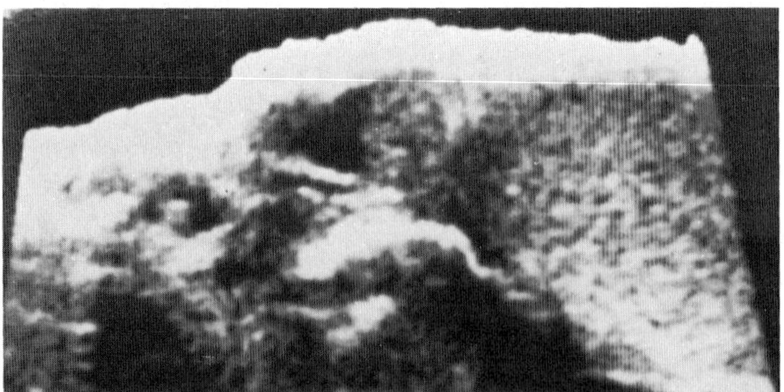

Fig. 2. Normal sonogram of the scrotum. The loose parenchyma of the testicle is well shown. The head of the epididymis sits on the top of the testicle in a cap-like fashion (left side)

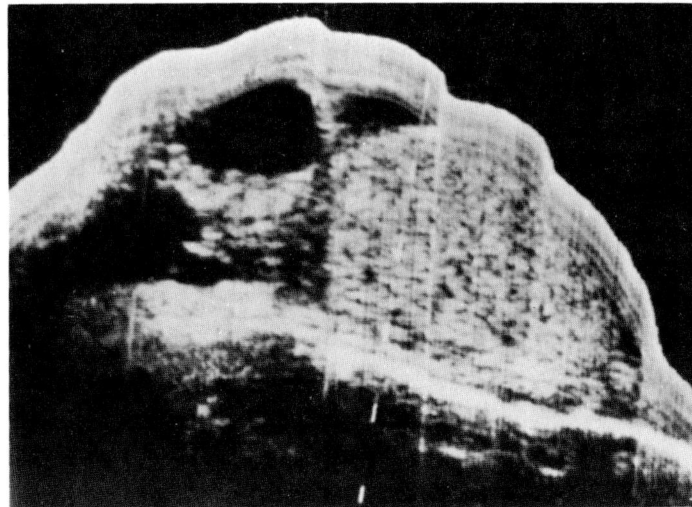

Fig. 3. Spermatocele: A large echolucent zone without a surrounding echogenic border. It is clearly delimited from the normal parenchyma of the testicle

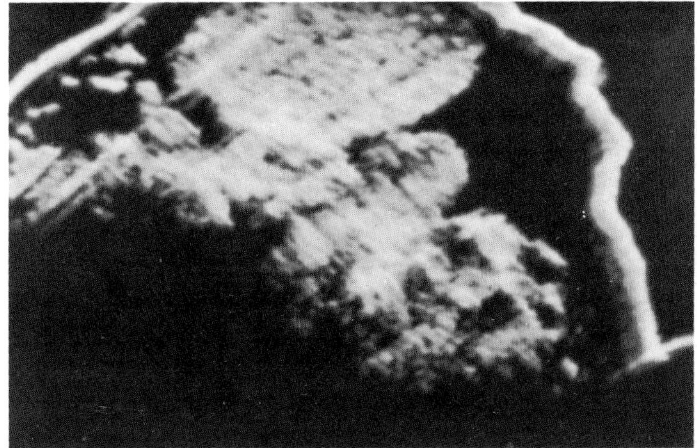

Fig. 4. Hydrocele and Varicocele: The echolucent fluid (dark areas) surrounds the testicle and the epididymis. The varicocele at the lower right shows the typical features: small echolucent zones with a surrounding echogenic border

The varicocele shows multiple, sonolucent zones with a surrounding echogenic border representing the vessel walls. A typical and unequivocal sonographic image of a varicocele is shown in Fig. 2.

The following diseases must be differentiated from this sonographic picture of a varicocele when the findings on palpation and inspection are equivocal.

A spermatocele (Fig. 3) shows one or more cystic areas, however, without the typical border of vessel walls. The cystic changes are located mainly close to the

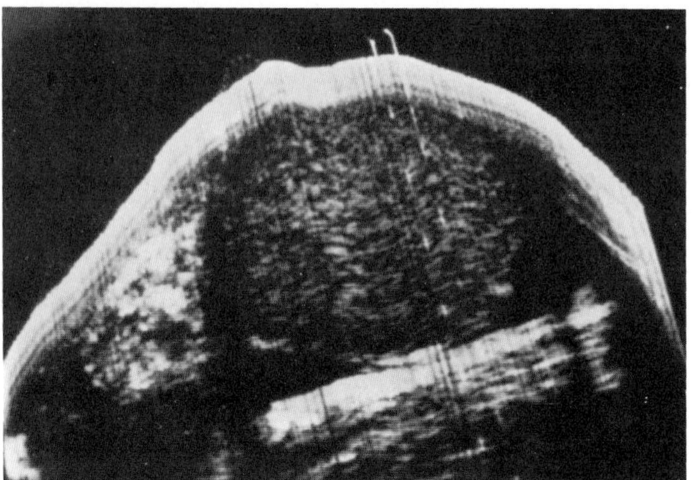

Fig. 5. Chronic epididymitis: The thickened head of the epididymis is shown to the right. It is on the top of the normal testicle

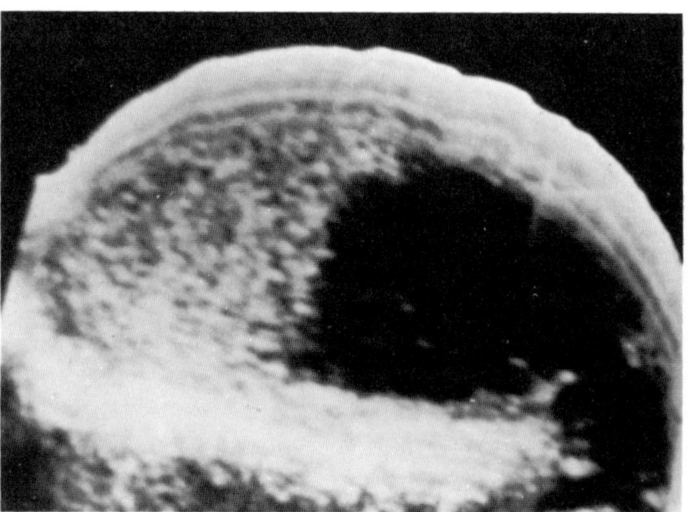

Fig. 6. Seminoma: A large echolucent mass in the upper part of the testicle can be seen (on the right)

head of the epididymis. Often multiple spermatoceles cannot be differentiated from a septated hydrocele. The diagnosis of a hydrocele poses no clinical or sonographic problem. Ultrasound, however, has the great advantage that it can clearly mark off the parenchyma of the testicle from the fluid of this scrotum.

Fig. 4 shows a hydrocele and a small varicocele as well. Chronic epididymitis is characterized by a thickening of the head of the epididymis without the typical echolucent zones of a varicocele (Fig. 5). In cases of doubt a repeat examination with the patient in an upright position reveals no changes.

A palpable testicular tumor presents a differential diagnostic problem to a varicocele. The sonographic picture of a testicular tumor shows a destruction of the homogeneous parenchymal pattern by an area of echolucency without the sonographic sign of a cyst (Fig. 6).

Summary

Usually a varicocele can clearly be differentiated from other scrotal masses by ultrasound because of the echolucent zones in the area of the testicle and the epididymis. Characteristically, there is a delicate surrounding echogenic border. Ultrasound is not necessary in the presence of unequivocal clinical findings of a varicocele.

However, if there is any doubt on palpation or if there is a suspicion of an additional disease of the scrotal contents, ultrasound is indicated, especially because no harmful side effects are known in diagnostic ultrasound.

References

1. Liebeskind D, Bases R, Elquin F, Neubort S, Leifer R, Goldberg R, Koenigsberg M (1979) Diagnostic Ultrasound: Effects on the DNA and Growth Patterns of Animal Cells. Radiol 131:177
2. Kucera H, Reinold E (1977) Über die Wirkung von Ultraschall auf die Mobilität menschlicher Spermien. Igls (Tirol): 7. Wissenschaftliche Gemeinschaftstagung der Deutschen und Österreichischen Gesellschaft zum Studium der Fertilität und Sterilität
3. Miskin, Buckspan M, Bain J (1977) Ultrasonographie examination of scrotal masses. J Urol (Baltimore) 117:185
4. Staehler G, Gebauer A, Mellin HE (1978) Sonographische Untersuchungen bei Erkrankungen des Skrotalinhaltes. Urologe A 17:247
5. Staehler G, Gebauer A: Diagnostische Bedeutung der Sonographie beim Hodentumor. Vortrag auf der gemeinsamen Tagung der Österreichischen Gesellschaft für Urologie und der Bayerischen Urologenvereinigung vom 17. bis 19. 5. 1979 in Salzburg

Comparison Between Different Methods
for the Diagnosis of Varicocele

F. COMHAIRE, M. KUNNEN, M. VANDEWEGHE, and M. SIMONS

Introduction

Whereas the diagnosis of large (grade II or III) [1 a] varicoceles should not cause any problems, small varicoceles are often more difficult to detect on clinical palpation. In addition, some patients present reflux in the internal spermatic vein without palpable distension of the pampiniform plexus [1]. Such patients are diagnosed as having subclinical reflux or subclinical varicocele. Since reflux is the pathogenetic factor of the epididymotesticular dysfunction in both clinical and subclinical varicoceles, treatment should be the same in both types of patients.

In order to diagnose internal spermatic venous reflux, four "objective" techniques are available. The following three methods can be considered as screening techniques, being non-invasive and relatively simple: scrotal (tele)thermography, Doppler flow measurement, and testicular perfusion analysis using radioisotopes. The fourth technique, retrograde venography of the internal spermatic vein, is more invasive and time consuming, and should be reserved for selected cases.

We have evaluated the different screening methods, bearing in mind the two following questions :

1. What is the value of the method for the selection of patients to undergo retrograde venography?
2. What is the accuracy of the method for the recognition of the side on which the reflux occurs?

Techniques and Results

Comparison Between Measurement of Scrotal Perfusion Using Radioisotope and Telethermography

The estimation of testicular perfusion with technetium has been used since 1973 for the differential diagnosis between testicular torsion and orchitis [2, 4]. Recently the technique has been explored for the detection of varicocele.

First, the thyroid is blocked by oral administration of 200 mg sodium perchlorate; an i.v. bolus of 10 mcurie sodium pertechnetate is then injected. With the patient standing erect, the radioactivity over the pelvic region and scrotum is recorded by means of a gamma camera. Eight registrations are made at 4 s intervals, followed by one summation registration covering the period from 30 to 120 s after injection. In normal men the femoral and iliac veins are clearly visible, whereas little radioactivity is registered over the scrotal region, in which the activity is symmetrically distributed (Fig. 1).

Some patients with varicocele do present an increased radioactivity on the affected hemiscrotum (Fig. 2). This finding proves that blood containing radioactive technetium stagnates in the scrotal venous plexus.

The method induces a testicular irradiation of no more than 110–120 mrad, i.e., about one-tenth of the irradiation inflicted by i.v. pyelography. The method is rapid and simple, and the patient does not even need to undress. However, in our hands, the method is not adequate for screening of subclinical varicocele.

A comparative study was performed in 51 men consulting for infertility. All were subjected to clinical examination, scrotal telethermography and, on the same day, testicular perfusion registration [6].

Thermography was positive in 12 of 13 cases with clinically palpable varicocele; in only 9 cases, however, was the technetium perfusion abnormal. Seven of 12 pa-

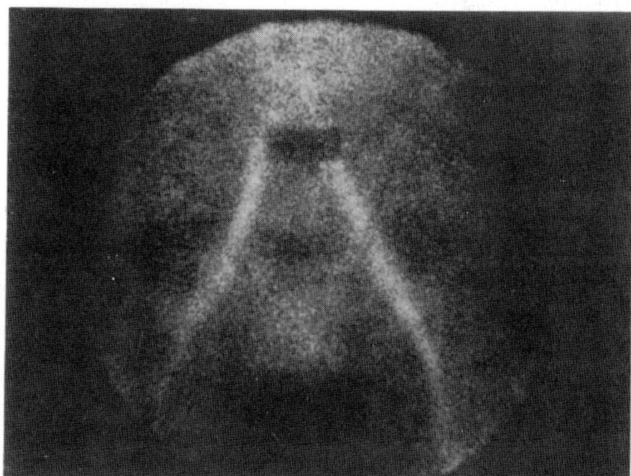

Fig. 1. Isotope scanning of the scrotum in a normal man without varicocele. There is a discrete retention of technetium symmetrically distributed over both sides of the scrotum

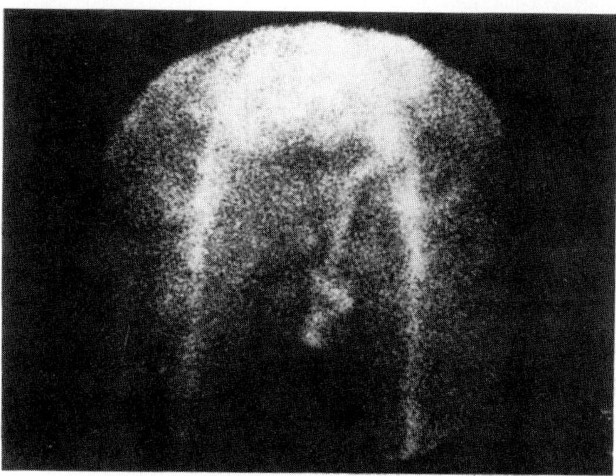

Fig. 2. Technetium scanning of the scrotum of a patient with left side varicocele. Stasis occurs of isotope-loaded blood in the distended pampiniform plexus

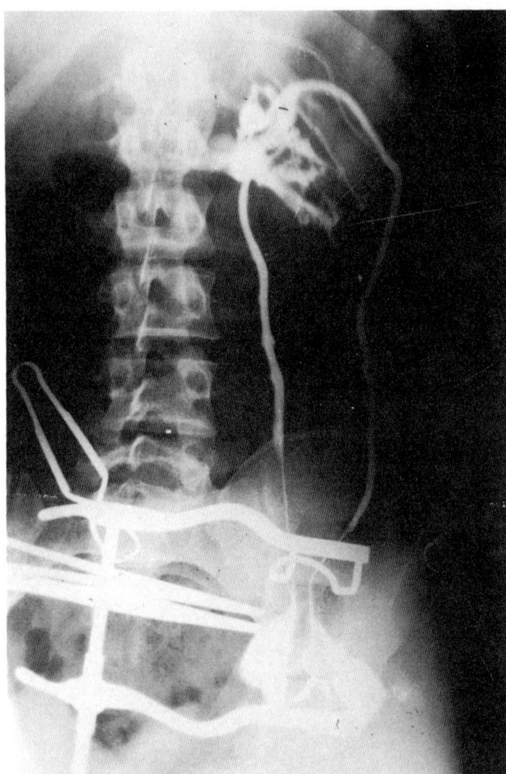

Fig. 3. *Ascending* venogram performed during surgery (Dept. of Urology, Dir. Prof. Dr. W. Desy) on a patient with palpable varicocele but (falsely) negative *retrograde* venogram. The internal spermatic vein presents two sets of valves in its paravertebral segment, which explains the absence of reflux on the retrograde venogram. Reflux occurs through a large bypass between a segmentary renal vein and the pampiniform plexus. The collateral bypass is situated at a rather remarkable distance from the spermatic vein, both joining together at the level of the internal inguinal ring

tients suspected of varicocele on clinical palpation presented a positive thermogram, as against only 2 with a positive perfusion study. Finally, of 26 cases clinically not suspected of varicocele, 4 had an abnormal thermographic registration, whereas in none was the technetium scan disturbed.

This comparison leads to the conclusion that technetium scanning certainly results in a rather large number of false negative registrations. Such patients do present spermatic venous reflux, as evidenced by means of thermography, but no stasis of blood seems to occur in the pampiniform plexus and therefore the technetium scan remains negative.

It is suggested that in these cases reflux is compensated through increased collateral efflux along the cremasteric and deferential veins.

Comparison Between Palpation, Doppler Flow Measurement, Telethermography, and Venography

The next comparative study concerns 81 patients in whom a retrograde venography of the internal spermatic vein was performed during the year 1979. It should be stressed that the population under study is not an unselected group of men consulting for infertility.

Included are only those cases in which spermatic venous reflux was suspected on the basis of either clinical palpation and/or scrotal thermography and/or Doppler flow measurement.

Comparison Between Retrograde Venography and Clinical Examination. Phlebography revealed a retrograde opacification of the internal spermatic vein in 90% of cases. Two retrograde venograms were faulty negative; indeed, no retrograde opacification could be demonstrated, despite the presence of a clinically evident varicocele which was confirmed at operation. In one of these cases an ascending phlebogram was performed during surgery (performed using Bernardi's technique).

The varicocele appeared to be due to the presence of reflux in a large collateral vessel connecting to an intrarenal cranial ramification of the renal vein, whereas the proper internal spermatic vein ended in the renal vein at the usual place, but presented competent valves (Fig. 3).

Clinical Examination vs. Retrograde Phlebography. The clinical examination had correctly detected the varicocele in 56 of 81 cases (69%). In another nine cases reflux was suspected and confirmed by venography (Table 1). In the remaining 16 cases (20%), the clinical examination failed to detect reflux, which could, however, be demonstrated on the venogram.

As to the question whether the clinical examination had correctly localized the side at which the reflux occurred, only 29 of 162 sides (81×2) were misdiagnosed (Table 2). Commonly, simultaneous right side reflux occurring in a patient with left side varicocele remained undetected.

Comparison Between Doppler Flow Measurement and Retrograde Venography. The prediction made by the Doppler method, as far as detection of reflux is concerned,

Table 1. Comparison between palpation and venography

	No. of patients
Clinically positive	56 (69%)
Clinically doubtful	9 (11%)
Clinically negative	16 (20%)
	81

Table 2. Comparison between palpation and venography with regard to localization

Correct		133 (82%)
False negative	left side	6
	right side	10
False positive	left side	9
	right side	4
		162

was correct in 31 of 38 cases (82%). In three cases (8%) the Doppler result was falsely negative; in four cases (10%) the Doppler examination suggested reflux which could not be confirmed by venography (Table 3).

As to the localization of reflux, the Doppler technique was fully correct in only 22 of 38 cases (58%). Falsely positive left side predictions and falsely negative right side predictions were particularly common (Table 4). It is possible that the number of falsely negative results may be reduced by the performance of a second examination with the patient in an upright position if the registration was negative in recumbent position.

Comparison Between Thermography and Venography. In 83% of 37 cases the indication for venography was correctly made on the basis of a positive scrotal thermogram. Falsely positive recordings occurred in five patients (14%); a falsely negative result was obtained in only one case (3%) (Table 5).

Table 3. Comparison between Doppler and thermography

	No. of patients
Doppler correct	31 (82%)
False negative	3 (8%)
False positive	4 (10%)
	38

Table 4. Comparison between Doppler and venography with regard to localization

Doppler Correct		59 (78%)
False negative	left side	3
	right side	5
False positive	left side	7
	right side	2
		76

Table 5. Comparison between thermography and venography

	No. of patients
Thermography correct	31 (83%)
False negative	1 (3%)
False positive	5 (14%)
	37

Table 6. Comparison between thermography and venography with regard to localization

Thermography		
Correct		62 (84%)
False negative	left side	2
	right side	4
False positive	left side	4
	right side	2
		74

Table 7. Comparison between Doppler and thermography

Both correct		16 (76%)
False negative	Doppler	1[a]
	thermo-	2[b]
False positive	Doppler	1
	thermo-	1
		21

[a] Proven upon venography
[b] In one case proven upon venography

As to the precision of the thermography in regard to the prediction of localization of reflux, this was correct in 27 of 37 cases (73%). In the remaining 20% of cases both false negative and false positive recordings occurred, both at the left and at the right side (Table 6).

Comparison Between Doppler Flow Measurement and Thermography

In an additional group of 21 men with infertility (not included in the previous studies), both Doppler flow measurement and scrotal telethermography were performed. Not all of these patients were subjected to retrograde venography (Table 7). In 16 patients (76%) the result of both examinations was identical: 8 times both were positive, 8 times both were negative. In three cases (14%) the Doppler method suggested reflux, whereas the thermogram was normal. In the first of these three cases the venogram was positive, confirming the Doppler result. In the second case the clinical palpation was convincingly positive, whereas in the third no varicocele could be detected on palpation.

In two cases (10%) the inverse occurred: the Doppler measurement was negative, whereas the thermogram clearly indicated the presence of reflux. One patient indeed had reflux on the venogram; in the other case the clinical palpation was negative.

This comparison suggests that both methods are about equivalent.

Discussion

The results of the studies reported here appear to be less favorable than those reported previously [1], the percentage of correct predictions by means of the screening technique tending to be lower. This is mainly due to the selection of cases. The study group (see p 91) consisted of men suspected of varicocele and in whom a retrograde venography was considered to be indicated. If we had included those cases in which no varicocele was suspected clinically, and in which the screening examinations had resulted in negative findings and therefore were not subjected to venography, the percentage of correct predictions would probably have been higher. It is estimated that less than 5% of such overall negative cases unexpectedly present reflux on the venogram.

In our opinion it is not justified (both for ethical and for practical reasons) to perform a retrograde venography in all patients with unexplained infertility. Such exploration has, however, been performed and yielded unsuspected reflux in 40% to 50% of the patients examined by venography [5]. Jecht et al. [3] could demonstrate reflux in the left spermatic vein in 28 out of 54 patients with reduced semen quality but no evidence of clinical varicocele. After preselection of the patients through screening methods, the percentage of positive venograms increases to 90%.

Systematic screening of infertile patients for the presence of (subclinical) varicocele appears to be useful for the following reasons:

1. For the elimination of patients most probably not having reflux. Personal experience as well as data reported by others indicate that, if both clinical palpation and scrotal thermography are negative, reflux is very uncommon.
2. For the selection of patients with subclinical varicocele or as an aid in the diagnosis of patients with doubtful clinical findings. In our study group, 24% of patients were correctly suspected to have subclinical varicocele on the basis of the results of the screening methods. In 5% of cases the suspicion was not confirmed by the retrograde venography (Table 8).

Table 8. Summary of results (in %) using different techniques

n	Palpation 81	Doppler 38	Thermography 37	Venography 81
Correct	69	82	83	97
False negative	(11)+20	8	3	3
False positive	0	10	14	0

Table 9. Summary of results (in %) using different techniques with regard to localization

n	Palpation 162	Doppler 76	Thermography 74
Correct	82	78	84
False negative	10	10	8
False positive	8	12	8

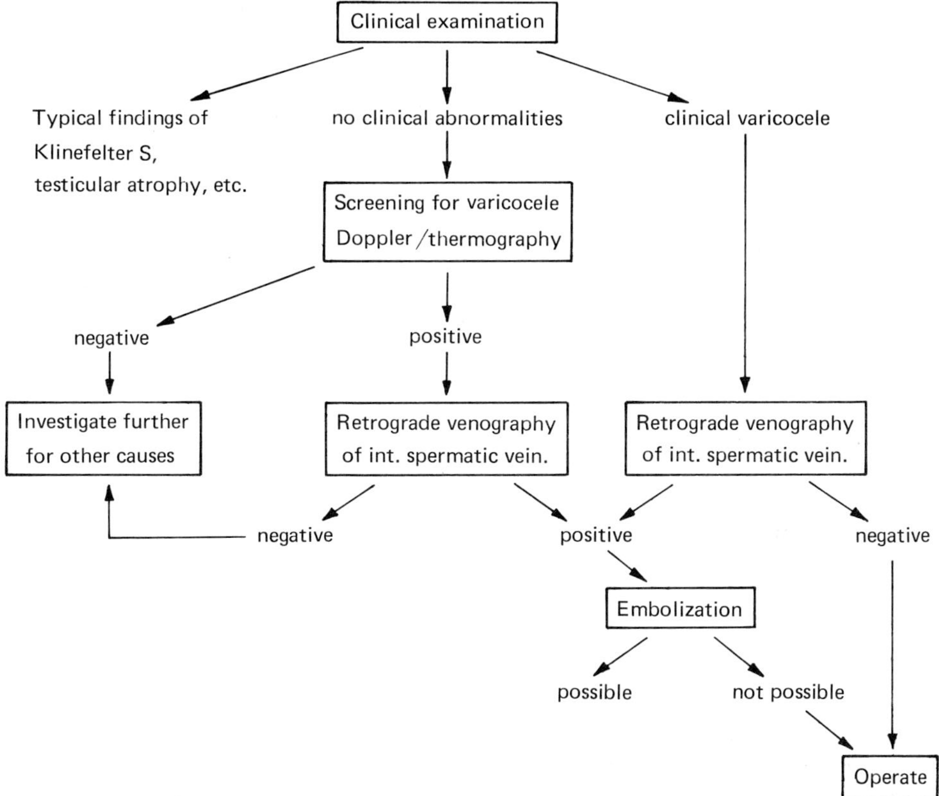

Fig. 4. Flow chart regarding diagnostic management in cases of male sub- and infertility

As far as the management of patients with unexplained infertility is concerned, our study further suggests the following conclusions:

3. Doppler flow measurement and (tele)thermography appear to be equally efficient diagnostic tools (Table 8). The percentage of false negative Doppler results can probably be reduced by repeating the examination while the patient is in a standing position, if the result in recumbent position is negative or inconclusive. Telethermography seems to permit a somewhat more accurate prediction of the side of reflux; however, the Doppler equipment is cheaper and easier to manipulate. At the moment the Doppler method seems more suitable for wide spread use; however, comparative studies using the cheaper equipment for contact thermography should be encouraged.
4. It seems unacceptable to decide whether surgical intervention should be unilateral, at either the left or right side, or bilateral, based on only the results of the screening techniques. In our opinion, retrograde venography remains necessary before an operation is performed (Table 9).

In summary, the flow chart shown in Fig. 4 is suggested for the diagnostic management of patients with varicocele or with unexplained infertility.

References

1. Comhaire F, Monteyne R, Kunnen M (1976) The value of scrotal thermography as compared with selective retrograde venography of the internal spermatic vein for the diagnosis of "subclinical" varicocele. Fertil Steril 27:694–698
1a. Dubin L, Amelar RD (1970) Varicocele size and results of varicocelectomy in selected subfertile men with varicocele. Fertil Steril 21:606–609
2. Holder LE, Martire JR, Holmes ER, Wagner HN (1977) Testicular radionuclide angiography and static imaging: anatomy, scintigraphic interpretation, and clinical indications. Radiology 125:739–752
3. Jecht E, Zeitler E, Herzinger R (1980) Die subklinische Varikozele. In: Schirren C, Mettler L, Semm K (Hrsg) Fortschritte der Fertilitätsforschung 8. Grosse, Berlin, pp 323–326
4. Nadel NS, Gitter MH, Hahn LC et al. (1973) Preoperative diagnosis of testicular torsion. Urology 1:478–479
5. Schellen AMCH, Hardy GH (1978) Phlebography, an important diagnostic tool in the work-up of the subfertile or infertile male. Ann of the group for the study of fertility, vol 5, part II, Antwerpen, pp 1–3
6. Vandeweghe M, Comhaire F, Simons M (1978) Investigation of the testicular blood circulation with technesium; first evaluation of the diagnostic usefulness. Ann of the group for the study of fertility, vol 5, part II, Antwerpen, pp 13–16

IV. Endocrinology and Immunology

Hormone Levels and Sperm Counts in Patients with Varicocele

H. Niermann, A. T. Harahap, and P. M. Kövary

It is well known that fertility may be significantly impaired in patients with varicocele. Surgical treatment is generally recommended. The incidence of varicocele among patients referred to fertility clinics has been reported to range between 4.6% [10] and 39% [4]. A recent review covering 20 362 patients from nine different fertility clinics revealed an incidence of 11.7% [20]. Among 10 000 patients attending our clinic, varicocele was observed in 15%. Surgeons may hesitate to perform the operation, since even in patients with large varicocele, normozoospermia may be found [7, 13, 15, 18] and oligo- or azoospermia may be associated with slight varicocele [8].

In the study described below, hormone levels were measured in untreated and treated patients with varicocele. The results confirm earlier reports indicating that in patients with varicocele there may not only be a disturbance of exocrine but also of endocrine testicular functions. Since improvement of seminal quality occurred in most treated patients, surgical treatment is recommended.

Methods

Semen and hormone analyses were performed in 32 patients with very large varicocele, in 36 patients with medium-size varicocele, and in 24 patients with minimum expression of the disease [2]. Postoperative investigations were performed in 14 patients.

Basal plasma LH, FSH, and testosterone levels (10°° a.m.) were measured by radioimmunoassay with commercially available reagents (Serono, Freiburg, Federal Republic of Germany).

Results

Pre-operative Findings

The results of pre-operative sperm counts and hormone levels are summarized in Table 1. LH was slightly elevated in 16 patients; FSH was slightly raised in only four patients.

Table 1. Plasma LH, FSH, and testosterone levels and sperm counts in patients with varicocele

Varicocele	n	LH (mIU/ml)		FSH (mIU/ml)		Testosterone (ng/ml)		Sperm count	
		$\bar{x}$	SD	$\bar{x}$	SD	$\bar{x}$	SD	mill/ml	SD
Very large	32	5.5	4.1	6.2	2.2	5.3	2.1	22.0	15.3
Medium-sized	36	6.5	3.2	6.4	2.5	6.2	1.9	13.0	7.2
Slight	24	7.2	4.3	6.9	3.1	6.9	2.2	9.7	18.0
Normal		5 – 10		3 – 12		4 – 9		40 mill/ml	

Postoperative Findings

In 12 of 14 treated patients, an increase of the sperm count (1.5–3.2) could be achieved. Plasma gonadotropin levels were normal in all patients. Testosterone levels were subnormal (3–4 ng/ml) in six of the treated patients.

Discussion

An inverse relationship between the clinical expression of varicocele and the sperm count was observed in the untreated patients. It appears that the size of varicocele does not provide prognostic help. Early investigators were reluctant to perform varicocele operations, since they did not see beneficial effects [9]. It may still be difficult to convince surgeons to perform the operation, although the sperm counts tend to increase in most patients after surgical treatment [1, 3, 4, 5, 6, 18, 19, 21].

Urinary FSH excretion (measured by passive hemagglutination) was found to be negatively correlated with the sperm count in patients with varicocele [14]. This may indicate functional impairment of spermiogenesis. Varicocele may lead primarily to testicular damage which, by feedback mechanisms, causes an increase of FSH [14]. Elevated plasma FSH levels were also demonstrable by the more sensitive radioimmunoassay [23]. In the latter study, 6 of 40 patients with varicocele had elevated FSH levels. Although an improvement of the seminal quality could be achieved by surgical treatment, plasma FSH levels remained elevated after the operation in four patients. In our study, however, increased FSH levels were not demonstrable.

While we could not correlate the degree of varicocele to seminal quality, plasma testosterone levels tended to be lower in patients with a more expressed varicocele. LH levels were not influenced. Also, in patients who had received surgical treatment, LH levels were normal. The finding of subnormal testosterone levels in 6 of 14 treated patients remains unexplained. An impairment of Leydig cell function in varicocele patients is known from various studies, although conflicting results have also been reported [11, 12]. Histologically, tubular atrophy, peritubular fibrosis, vascular alterations, and Leydig cell hyperplasia have been reported [7]. These were attributed to disturbed testicular blood flow in patients with varicocele [7]. Gonadotropins were normal in 504 patients with varicocele, but treatment with HCG improved seminal quality, indicating impaired Leydig cell function [3]. From seminal fructose levels it had been concluded that Leydig cell function remains preserved [11]. However, normal seminal fructose levels can no longer be accepted as a criterion for intact Leydig cell function. In an early study, plasma testosterone levels of 37 patients with varicocele were lower than testosterone levels in 65 control patients [16]. Other authors have confirmed this observation [17, 22].

References

1. Charny CW (1962) Effect of varicocele on fertility. Fertil Steril 13:47–56
2. Dubin L, Amelar RD (1970) Varicocele size and results of varicocelectomy in selected subfertile men with varicocele. Fertil Steril 21:606–609
3. Dubin L, Amelar RD (1975) Varicocelectomy as therapy in male infertility: A study of 504 cases. Fertil Steril 26:217–220
4. Dubin L, Amelar RD (1971) Etiologic factors in 1.294 consecutive cases of male infertility. Fertil Steril 22:469–474
5. Fernando N, Leonard JM, Paulsen CA (1976) The role of varicocele in male infertility. Andrologia 8:1–9
6. Haensch R (1976) Der Einfluß der Varikozelenoperation nach Palomo auf das Spermiogramm. Hautarzt 27:449–452
7. Haensch R, Hornstein O (1968) Varicocele und Fertilitätsstörung. Dermatologica 136:335–349
8. Jecht E, Herzinger R, Zeitler E (1980) Die subklinische Varikozele. Grosse, Berlin, pp 323–326 (Fortschr Fertil Forschg, vol 8)
9. Klika M (1958) Die Unzulänglichkeit der chirurgischen Therapie der idiopathischen Varikozele. Z Urol 51:633–639
10. Klosterhalfen H, Schirren C (1964) Über die operative Wiederherstellung der Zeugungsfähigkeit des Mannes. Dtsch Med Wochenschr 89:2234–2241
11. Ludwig C, Jentzsch R, Peters HJ (1974) Fertilität bei idiopathischer Varikozele. Fortschr Med 92:1233–1278
12. Lunglmayr G (1978) Operative Aspekte der Therapie der männlichen Fertilität in: Physiologie und Pathophysiologie der Hodenfunktion, Senge, Th, Neumann F, Schenck B (eds). Thieme, Stuttgart, pp 132–141
13. MacLeod J (1965) Seminal cytology in the presence of varicocele. Fertil Steril 16:735–757
14. Mauss J, Schach H, Scheidt J (1974) Andrologische Untersuchungen bei subfertilen Männern vor und nach Varicocelenoperation. Hautarzt 25:394–398
15. Niermann H (1960) Ergebnisse der Untersuchung von 2000 Patienten mit Fertilitätsstörungen. Arch Klin Exp Dermatol 211:156–160
16. Raboch J, Starka L (1971) Androgene und koitale Aktivität von Patienten mit Varikozele. Grosse, Berlin (Fortschr Fertil Forschg, vol 2, pp 141–144)
17. Rodriguez-Rigau LJ, Weiss DB, Zukerman Z, Grotjan HE, Smith KD, Steinberger E (1978) A possible mechanism for the determinal effect of varicocele on testicular function in man. Fertil Steril 30:577–585
18. Schirren C, Klosterhalfen H (1966) Die Spermatogenese bei Varikozele. Z Hautkr 20:372–377
19. Scott LS, Young D (1962) Varicocele: A study of its effects of human spermatogenesis, and of the results produced by spermatic vein ligation. Fertil Steril 13:325–334
20. Steeno O, Knops J, Declerck L, Adimoelja A, van de Yorde H (1976) Prevention of fertility disorders by detection and treatment of varicocele at school and college age. Andrologia 8:47–53

21. Tulloch WS (1952) A consideration of sterility factors in the light of subsequent pregnancies. Edinburgh Med J 59:29
22. Weiss DP, Rodriguez-Rigau L, Smith KD, Chowdhury A, Steinberger E (1978) Quantitation of leydig cells in testicular biopsies of oligospermic men with varicocele. Fertil Steril 30:305–312
23. Wichmann U, Krause W, Weidner W (1980) Der Wert der Hormonbestimmung in der Prognose der Varicocele. Grosse, Berlin (Fortschr Fertil Forschg, vol 8), pp 191–193

Testosterone in Peripheral Plasma, Spermatic Veins, and Testicular Tissue of Patients with Varicocele

H.-J. VOGT, K. M. PIRKE, and R. SINTERMANN

It is generally believed that a varicocele impairs tubular function and spermatogenesis. It is, however, unclear whether or not the Leydig cell function also decreases. Raboch and Stárka [7] observed testosterone concentrations in plasma that were half as high in patients with varicocele than in healthy controls. In contrast, Swerdloff and Walsh [9] found normal testosterone concentrations. This was confirmed by Comhaire and Vermeulen [3], who found normal testosterone in all patients with varicocele. One-third of their patients, however, complained of erectile impotence. This subgroup had testosterone concentrations in the lower part of the normal range. Concentrations increased after surgery, together with an improvement of the impotence. We studied the testosterone concentrations in peripheral plasma in the spermatic vein, and in testicular tissue of patients with varicocele in order to further investigate the problem of Leydig cell function in patients with varicocele.

Patients

Twenty-eight patients aged 17–40 years were studied. Except for one patient, the varicocele was on the left side. Only two patients suffered from erectile impotence. Peripheral blood was taken on the day before surgery between 10 and 12 a.m. In 18 patients, blood was obtained from the spermatic vein during the operation. A small catheter was inserted into the spermatic vein and 2–5ml blood was collected. In 10 patients a piece of testicular tissue (2–10 mg) was obtained by biopsy. The serum and the tissue samples were immediately frozen and kept at $-30\,°C$ until analyzed.

Several control groups of patients and normal subjects were studied for reasons of comparison. Fifty normal, healthy men studied earlier in our laboratory [5] served as a control group for testosterone in peripheral plasma. For obvious reasons, blood from the spermatic vein cannot be obtained from healthy subjects. We obtained blood from the spermatic vein in 13 patients who suffered from carcinoma of the prostate and were castrated for therapeutic reasons [6]. These patients were between 60 and 81 years old.

As the control group for the intratesticular testosterone concentrations, we studied a group of 45 infertile patients aged 18–40 years who underwent diagnostic biopsy of the testes. This group was further characterized earlier [6].

Methods

Testosterone in peripheral plasma was measured by radioimmunoassay without chromatographic separation as described earlier [4]. Testosterone in the spermatic vein plasma was measured by radioimmunoassay, including thin-layer chromatography [4]. Fifty microliters of the 1:20 diluted serum were used in the assay.

Testicular tissue was homogenized in 1 ml isotonic phosphate buffer pH 7.4 in an all-glass Potter homogenizer. Between 25 and 200 µl of the homogenate were analyzed in the assay.

Results and Discussion

Testosterone in peripheral plasma is listed in Table 1. As can be seen, there is no difference between the patients with varicocele and the normal subjects. This finding is in agreement with the data of Swerdloff and Walsh [9]. In contrast to Comhaire and Vermeulen, we did not find a group of patients with varicocele who had testosterone values in the lower normal range and who complained of erectile impotence. Among our patients there were only two who complained of impotence. Both had testosterone values in the middle of the normal range. We studied ten patients with varicocele 3 weeks to 10 months after surgery. These patients had testosterone

Table 1. Testosterone in peripheral plasma of patients with varicocele and in the control groups

	Testosterone		Age	
	Mean value (ng/100 ml)	Range (ng/100 ml)	Mean value (years)	Range (years)
Varicocele ($n=28$)	598	340 – 988	28	17 – 40
Normal healthy subjects ($n=50$)	545	315 – 965	28	19 – 54
Infertile patients ($n=45$)	562	325 – 943	27	18 – 40
Patients with carcinoma of the prostate ($n=23$)	391	198 – 825	77	60 – 93

Table 2. Testosterone in the spermatic vein of patients with varicocele and with carcinoma of the prostate

		Varicocele	Prostate carcinoma
Testosterone (μg/liter)	$\overline{X}$	229	272
	Range	29 – 381	130 – 508
Gradient spermatic/ peripheral plasma	$\overline{X}$	49.4	73.5
	Range	8.7 – 87.2	40.5 – 139.2

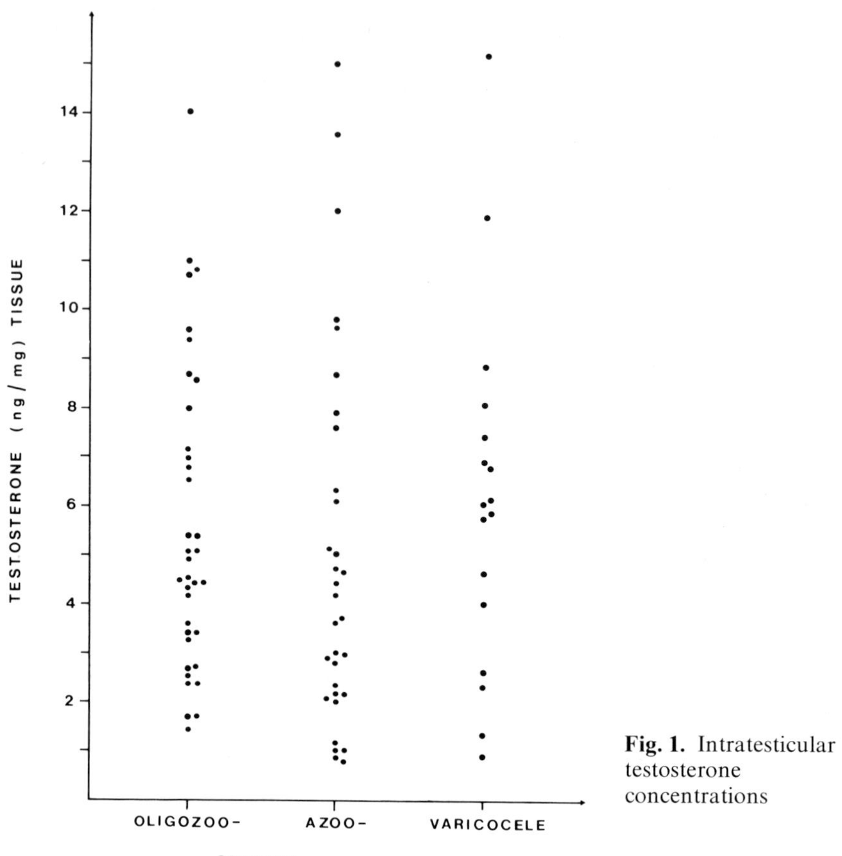

Fig. 1. Intratesticular testosterone concentrations

levels between 450 and 800 ng/100 ml (average, 586) before the operation and between 450 and 875 ng/100 ml (average, 614) afterwards. The slight increase of 4.7% was not significant. The difference between our finding and that of Comhaire and Vermeulen [3] cannot be explained at the moment. We may, however, speculate that the age of the patients explains the difference. Comhaire and Vermeulen's 10 patients with low testosterone and sexual insufficiency were 43 years old on average. In contrast, all our patients were younger than 40 years. It may well be, therefore, that in patients with varicocele there is a decrease in Leydig cell function already in the middle of life, while in normal subjects this decrease occurs only in the sixth and seventh decades [5, 10].

In Table 2, the testosterone levels in the spermatic vein of patients with varicocele and with a carcinoma of the prostate are listed. There was no significant difference between both groups. The range, however, was greater in the patients with varicocele. As can be seen in Table 1, the testosterone in the peripheral plasma of the older patients was much lower than in the younger patients and controls. This reflects the age-dependent decrease of testosterone, which is also seen in healthy old men [5]. Since the testosterone metabolism in old men is even slower than in young men [8], the fall in plasma testosterone indicates the decreased testosterone secretion in the old patients. We would therefore expect higher testosterone levels in the spermatic vein of young patients than of old patients. In contrast, we found no difference. The gradient from spermatic vein to peripheral plasma was, however, twice as high in old as in young patients with varicocele. We believe that the venous reflux from the renal vein into the spermatic vein, which was demonstrated by Ahlberg et al. [1] and by Charney and Baum [2], brings about a dilution of the spermatic vein blood and thus causes relatively low testosterone concentrations.

Figure 1 shows the intratesticular testosterone concentrations in patients with a varicocele and patients with oligozoospermia and azoospermia whom we have previously described [6]. In all groups there is a wide variability of tissue concentrations. The values are not lower in the patients with varicocele than in the infertile patients who were, as can be seen in Table 1, all normogonadotrophic.

In conclusion, measurement of testosterone in peripheral plasma, in the spermatic vein, and in testicular tissue of patients with varicocele did not reveal any evidence for an impaired Leydig cell function in patients younger than 40 years.

References

1. Ahlberg NE, Bartley O, Chidekel N, Fritjofsson A (1966) Phlebography in varicocele scroti. Acta Radiol [Diagn] 4:529–538
2. Charney CW, Baum S (1968) Varicocele and infertility. JAMA 204:1165–1168
3. Comhaire F, Vermeulen A (1975) Plasma testosterone in patients with varicocele and sexual inadequacy. J Clin Endocrinol 40:824–829
4. Pirke KM (1973) A comparison of three methods of measuring testosterone in plasma: competitive protein binding, radioimmunoassay without and radioimmunoassay including thin layer chromatography. Acta Endocrinol (Copenh) 74:168–176
5. Pirke KM, Doerr P (1973) Age-related changes and interrelationships between plasmia testosterone, oestradiol and testosterone-binding globulin in normal adult males. Acta Endocrinol (Copenh) 74:792
6. Pirke KM, Vogt H-J, Lehnig W, Sintermann R (1979) Intratesticular testosterone concentration in patients with disturbed fertility. Andrologia 11:320–325
7. Raboch J, Stárka L (1971) Hormonal testicular activity in men with a varicocele. Fertil Steril 22:152
8. Rubens H, Dhont M, Vermeulen A (1974) Further studies on Leydig cell function in old age. J Clin Endocrinol 39:40–45
9. Swerdloff RS, Walsh PC (1975) Pituitary and gonadal hormones in patients with varicocele. Fertil Steril 26:1006
10. Vermeulen A, Rubens R, Verdonck AL (1972) Testosterone secretion and metabolism in male senescence. J Clin Endocrinol 34:730

Varicocele Operation and Endocrine Parameters

E. W. Jecht and D. Brandl

In spite of a recent sceptical report [7], a beneficial effect of varicocele operation – commonly referred to as high ligation – on semen quality in patients with a varicocele appears to be established [for review see 4, 11]. The question of whether the postoperative improvement of sperm count is mirrored by a corresponding change of FSH has been studied by Schiff et al. [9]. They measured FSH as well as LH and testosterone in five patients with a varicocele and reduced semen quality prior to and 3 months following high ligation [9]. While there was a postoperative improvement in semen quality, no change was seen postoperatively for FSH, LH, and testosterone before and after stimulation with GnRH. However, the data of Schiff et al. [9] appear somewhat provisional due to the small number of patients and the relatively short time interval between operation and postoperative endocrine evaluation.

Eighteen patients (age 22–47 years, mean 32 years) with a left-sided clinical varicocele and reduced semen quality underwent high ligation of the left internal spermatic vein [technique of Bernardi (1)]. Shortly before and at different time intervals after the operation (mean 8.8 months, range 3–17 months), FSH, LH, and testosterone were measured in plasma prior to and following intravenous injection of 100 µg GnRH[1]. The methods for the hormone assays have been reported previously [6]. Semen analyses [5] were performed simultaneously with the hormone determinations. For statistical analysis, the Wilcoxon matched-pairs signed-ranks test [10] was employed.

There was almost no difference between the pre- and the postoperative values of FSH (Fig. 1). In contrast, LH (Fig. 2) was significantly higher after operation both before ($P < 0.05$) and following ($P < 0.01$) stimulation with GnRH. The values of testosterone showed a tendency to prestimulatory lower values after operation and were significantly lower ($P < 0.05$) 180 min following stimulation with GnRH (Fig. 3). No change was seen postoperatively for any of the seminal parameters.

Our results confirm the findings of Schiff et al. [9] for FSH, showing no change following operation. Semen quality, on the other hand, improved in the patients of Schiff et al. [9] but not in our patients. The lack of a postoperative change in FSH for our patients corresponds well with the lack of improvement in semen quality. This cannot be said from the data of Schiff et al. in which a reactive decrease of (poststimulatory elevated) FSH would have been consistent with the improvement of sperm count. The simultaneous postoperative decrease of testosterone and in-

---

1 Kindly donated by Hoechst AG

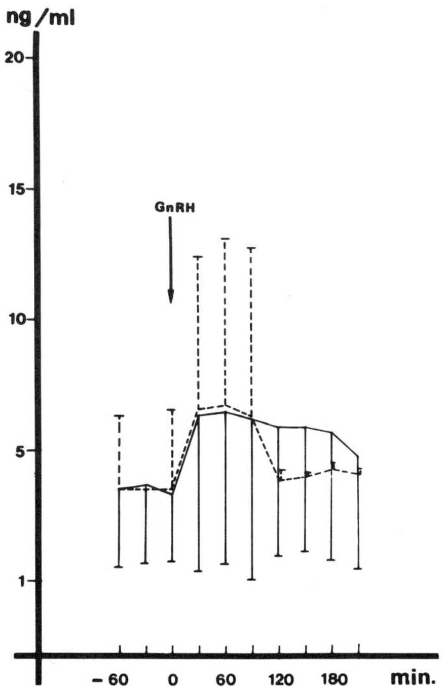

Fig. 1. Response of plasma FSH to stimulation with 100 µg GnRH before (———) and after (– – – –) high ligation (x̄±SD) (last four values postoperatively determined in five patients only)

Fig. 2. Response of plasma LH to stimulation with 100 µg GnRH before (———) and after (– – – –) high ligation (x̄±SD)

crease of LH in our patients present an unexpected finding and contrast with the lack of change found by Schiff et al. [9]. Do the postoperative rise of LH and fall of testosterone reflect – or perhaps cause – the nonrespondence of semen quality to high ligation in our patients? Rodriguez-Rigau et al. [8] recently suggested an indirect action of varicocele on spermatogenesis mediated via depressed testosterone production due to impaired Leydig cell function. But why then should high ligation adversely affect Leydig cell function and, consequently, testosterone production in our patients?

Comhaire and Vermeulen [2] reported a postoperative increase of basal values of testosterone in 10 patients with a clinical varicocele. However, preoperative testosterone levels were low in these ten patients [2] while they were "normal" in our 18 patients.

Our results, apparently, pose more questions than they answer. If we assume a – possibly transient – impairment of Leydig cell function by high ligation, the increase of LH could be explained as a reaction of upper centers to the decreased testosterone production. As a result of the elevated LH, new Leydig cells could originate (neogenesis of Leydig cells, [3]) and eventually normalize the testosterone production at a later point in time. Sufficient testosterone levels, in turn, would create

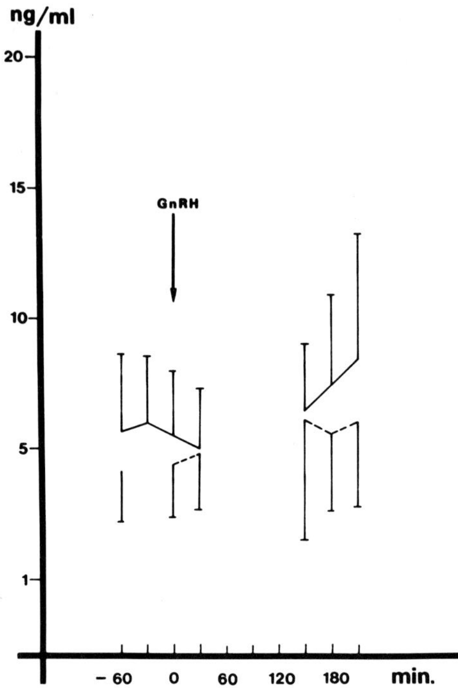

Fig. 3. Response of plasma testosterone to stimulation with 100 µg GnRH before (——) and after (– – – –) high ligation ($\bar{x}\pm$ SD) (values at 60, 90, and 120 min not determined)

more favorable conditions for spermatogenesis in the seminiferous tubules and thus lead to improved semen quality. In this scheme, the time factor could perhaps partly explain the disagreement between our data and the results of Schiff et al. [9] and of Comhaire and Vermeulen [2], respectively.

In conclusion, while the interpretation of our results remains highly speculative, the definite postoperative change of LH and testosterone may in time shed further light on the mechanism of varicocele action.

References

1. Bernardi R (1980) Varicocele. El Ateneo, Buenos Aires
2. Comhaire F, Vermeulen A (1975) Plasma testosterone in patients with varicocele and sexual inadequacy. J Clin Endocrinol 40:824
3. Hornstein O (1964) Zur Klinik und Histopathologie des männlichen primären Hypogonadismus. III. Hodenparenchymschäden durch Varicocelen. Arch Klin Exp Dermatol 218:347
4. Jecht E (1977) Varikozele und Fertilität. Z Haut Geschlechtskr 138:177
5. Jecht E, Kiessling W, Ude P (1979) Grundriß der Andrologie für die Praxis. Ichthyol-Gesellschaft, Hamburg
6. Jecht E, Klupp E, Heidler R, Huben H, Schwarz W (1980) Investigation of the hormonal axis hypothalamus – pituitary – gonads in 20 dialyzed men. Andrologia 12:146
7. Nilsson S, Edvinsson A, Nilsson B (1979) Improvement of semen and pregnancy rate after ligation and division of the internal spermatic vein: Fact or fiction? Br J Urol 51:591

 8. Rodriguez-Rigau LJ, Weiss DB, Zukerman Z, Grotjan H, Smith KD, Steinberger E (1978) A possible mechanism for the detrimental effect of varicocele on testicular function in man. Fertil Steril 30:577
 9. Schiff I, Wilson E, Newton R, Shane J, Kates R, Ryan KJ, Naftolin F (1976) Serum luteinizing hormone, follicle-stimulating hormone, and testosterone responses to gonadotropin-releasing factor in males with varicoceles. Fertil Steril 27:1059
10. Siegel S (1956) Nonparametric statistics for the behavioral sciences. McGraw-Hill, New York Toronto London
11. Verstoppen GR, Steeno OP (1977) Varicocele and the pathogenesis of the associated subfertility. A review of the various theories. II. Results of surgery. Andrologia 9:293

Hormonal Testicular Function in Patients with Varicocele

F. COMHAIRE and A. VERMEULEN

Physiopathology

Epididymal-testicular dysfunction in patients with varicocele is due to reflux of blood in the internal spermatic vein. We have demonstrated that this refluxing blood contains an elevated concentration of cathecholamines [3]. Recently, the concentrations of adrenaline and noradrenaline were measured by radioimmunoassay (Dr. Moerman, Heymans Institute, University Ghent) in spermatic venous blood of patients with varicocele during diagnostic phlebography (C. Bruijnen, unpublished observations).

With the patient in recumbent position, the mean concentration of noradrenaline particularly was only slightly more elevated in spermatic venous blood ($\bar{X} = 28$ ng/dliter) than in peripheral venous blood ($\bar{X} = 17$ ng/dliter). When the patient was moved to a standing position the spermatic venous concentration of noradrenaline increased to mean 44 ng/dliter, which is significantly higher than the peripheral concentration.

It is suggested that noradrenaline is transferred, by means of counter current exchange at the level of the pampiniform plexus, to the testicular arteries. This would result in chronic constriction of the intratesticular arterioles, causing decreased testicular perfusion. Indeed, a decreased testicular blood supply could be objectivated during the arterial phase of the perfusion examination after bolus i.v. injection of Technetium (C. Nahoum, personal communication). Furthermore, chronic exposure to increased cathecholamine concentrations might cause hyperplasia of the endothelial cells, as demonstrated in testicular arterioles of patients with varicocele [5, 8].

The impairment of testicular blood supply interferes with Sertoli cell function [5] and histology [8], resulting in progressive vacuolization of these cells and sloughing of spermatogenic cells.

Also, deficient arterial blood supply may cause Leydig cell deficiency.

Testosterone

In 1971 Raboch and Starka [7] reported plasma testosterone levels to be decreased in patients with varicocele; we confirmed this observation [4]. In our patient population we detected a significant correlation between decreasing testosterone concentration and increasing age. It is known that in normal men, mean peripheral testosterone concentration starts to decrease in the 6th or 7th decade. Patients with varicocele present such a decrease as early as the 4th and 5th decade. It is not clear whether this lower peripheral testosterone concentration is caused by a decreased testicular testosterone production or by decreased venous efflux.

In this last condition, the testosterone concentration in testicular tissue and spermatic venous blood should be normal. Recent measurements of testosterone in both testicular tissue [6] and in spermatic venous blood [9] indicate that decreased hormone production seems to occur in some varicocele cases, whereas in others a decreased venous return probably occurs.

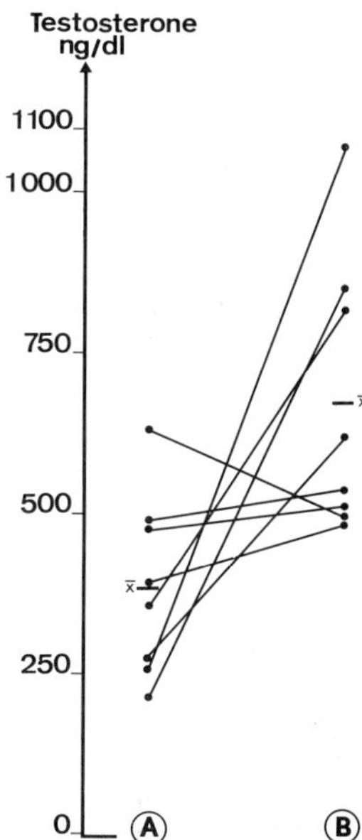

Fig. 1. Plasma testosterone concentrations in peripheral blood of eight patients with varicocele, before (**A**) and 3 months after (**B**) embolization of the internal spermatic vein with Bucrylate (M. Kunnen). The cases with a relatively low preoperative testosterone concentration present a significant increase, whereas the cases with normal preoperative concentration do not present significant changes

Regardless of the individual cause (whatever may be), as a result of their disease a number of patients with varicocele present a decreased peripheral testosterone concentration and this abnormality disappears after surgical correction [4]. Similarly, relatively low testosterone concentrations rapidly normalize after embolization of the internal spermatic vein (Fig. 1).

Hypothalamic Pituitary Function

Varicocele causes a demonstrable effect on the hypothalamo-pituitary-gonadal axes.

We performed preoperative LHRH tests in 23 patients with varicocele. In 13 of these patients, reevaluation was performed 3–6 months after surgical correction [1, 2]. The response to LHRH was evaluated by measuring the total secretion of LH and of FSH, as the sum Σ of LH and FSH values, 20, 40, and 60 min after i.v. injection of 400 µg LHRH.

Table 1. Relevant correlation between different testicular and pituitary parameters in 23 patients with varicocele before operation

	Σ LH	Σ FSH
Basal LH	0.37 $P < 0.1$	
Basal FSH		0.91 $P < 0.001$
Σ LH		0.82 $P < 0.001$
Sperm concentration	0.50 $P < 0.05$	0.46 $P < 0.05$
Plasma testosterone	0.38 $P < 0.1$	

The following correlations were found to be significant (Table 1):

1. Basal LH and basal FSH are significantly correlated to Σ LH and Σ FSH, respectively. For clinical purposes, one measurement of basal LH and FSH is therefore sufficient.
2. Values for Σ LH and Σ FSH are closely correlated. This may be due to either of the following possibilities:
   a) The feedback of pituitary LH and FSH secretion is regulated by one single substance.
   b) Pituitary feedback is regulated through two different substances, one secreted by the interstitial compartment regulating LH, and one from the tubular compartment regulating FSH. The varicocele disturbs both testicular compartments in a synchronous and parallel way.
3. The value for Σ FSH is inversely correlated with the sperm count. This could have been expected since inhibin, secreted by the Sertoli cells, is responsible for the FSH feedback, and also since the inhibin secretion will be reduced as Sertoli cell function is impaired and as spermatogenesis is disturbed.

Table 2. Relevant correlation between changes in different testicular and pituitary parameters in 13 patients before and after varicocele operation

	Σ LH	Σ FSH
Σ LH		0.58 $P < 0.1$
Sperm concentration	0.35 N.S.	0.74 $P < 0.05$
Plasma testosterone	0.09 N.S.	

4. A weak correlation was found between Σ LH and peripheral testosterone. The correlation between Σ LH and sperm count is statistically significant. Both LH and testosterone are secreted in pulses and present rapid and rather important physiological fluctuations within normal limits. Thus it could be expected that Σ LH and plasma testosterone would present, if anything, only a weak (inverse) correlation. More remarkable is the significant inverse correlation between Σ LH and sperm count. This suggests that a tubular factor (possibly also responsible for FSH feedback inhibition) interferes with the LH release in response to LHRH stimulation.

   After surgical cure of the varicocele, certain changes do occur in gonadal and pituitary function (Table 2).

5. After operation, Σ FSH presents changes correlated with the changes in sperm count. This observation proves that, after operation, tubular function improves, resulting in both increased sperm production and increased inhibin secretion. The latter produces a stronger inhibition of the pituitary FSH secretion. Since inhibin is secreted by the Sertoli cells, the results point to an improved Sertoli cell function after correction of the varicocele.

Conclusions

The disturbed spermatogenesis in patients with varicocele probably is due to disturbed Sertoli cell function. Sertoli cell insufficiency results in decreased sperm cell maturation and precocious sloughing of spermatogenic cells. At the same time, the inhibin secretion decreases, leading to an increased basal FSH concentration as well as an increased FSH response to LHRH.

Varicocele can also cause disturbance of Leydig cell function. This is evidenced by an age related, precocious decrease in peripheral testosterone concentration which can evoke a syndrome of "premature male climacteric".

The dysfunction of the Leydig cells can manifest itself in three different forms:

1. Low peripheral testosterone concentration together with a normal LH concentration. In these cases treatment of the varicocele always results in a normalization of the testosterone concentration.
2. Normal testosterone concentration with an increased LH level. This condition can be described as compensated Leydig cell insufficiency and is characterized by a decreased Leydig cell reserve. After treatment of the varicocele, LH normalizes in most of the patients.
3. Low peripheral testosterone concentration with increased LH concentration. This condition occurs in older patients or in cases with severe testicular damage (low testicular volume) and has a rather poor prognosis.

Finally, it appears that as far as the restitution of Leydig cell function is concerned, nonsurgical treatment by means of transcatheter embolization of the internal spermatic vein is as effective as surgical ligation.

References

1. Comhaire F (1976) Study of the hypothalamo-pituitary-testicular function in patients with varicocele before and after operation. Sperm Action. Prog Reprod Biol 1:187
2. Comhaire F, Dhondt M (1975) Influence of current modes of treatment in male infertility on the hypothalamo-pituitary testicular function. In: Schellen T (ed) Releasing factors and gonadotropic hormones in male and female sterility. European Press Medicon, part III, Ghent, p 117
3. Comhaire F, Vermeulen A (1974) Varicocele sterility: cortisol and cathecholamines. Fertil Steril 25:88
4. Comhaire F, Vermeulen A (1975) Plasma testosterone in patients with varicocele and sexual inadequacy. J Clin Endocrinol Metab 40:824
5. Hofman N, Hilscher B, . . . cf. MS 7 this volume pp 29 ff.
6. Pasqualini T, Chemes H, Coco R, Domené H, Campo S, Nicolau G, Lavieri J, Rivarola MA (1980) Testicular function in varicocele. Int J Androl 3:679–691
7. Raboch J, Starka L (1971) Hormonal testicular activity in men with a varicocele. Fertil Steril 22:152
8. Terquem A (1978) Etude ultrastructurale du testicule d'hommes porteurs de varicocele: résultats préliminaires. Contraception, Fertilité, Sexualité 6:599
9. de la Torre B, Noren S, Hedman M, Diczfalusy E (1978) Studies on the relationship between sperm count and steroid levels in the spermatic and cubital veins of patients with varicocele. Int J Androl 1:297

Enhanced Chemotactic Activity of Microphages in Varicocele

D. Djawari, K. H. Conrad, and E. W. Jecht

In 1977, we reported an increased phagocytotic activity in the semen of patients suffering from a varicocele. It was our assumption that this enhanced phagocytosis was caused by the varicocele [2].

In an attempt to confirm this assumption we compared the chemotactic activity of microphages from 23 patients with disturbed semen quality [3] and a clearly palpable varicocele and from 23 volunteers with normal semen analysis [3] and without a palpable varicocele.

Semen was collected by masturbation in sterile glass vials, and spermatozoa were separated from seminal plasma by gentle centrifugation. Employing a slightly modified Boyden technique, described elsewhere [1], we resuspended the spermatozoa in Hank's solution and incubated them together with autologous or homologous microphages (final concentration of spermatozoa 1×10^7/ml, of leukocytes 1×10^6/ml) in the chamber [1]. After incubation for three hours at 37 °C, the number of microphages migrating into the dividing filter was determined.

The number of immigrating microphages was clearly elevated when patients' leukocytes were incubated together with autologous spermatozoa (Fig. 1). In contrast, no chemotactic activity was detected for microphages from volunteers incubated with patients' spermatozoa (Fig. 2). When spermatozoa from volunteers were ex-

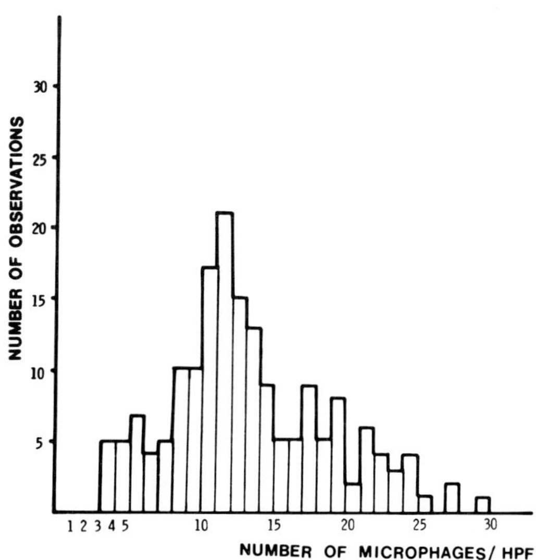

Fig. 1. Patients' spermatozoa incubated with autologous microphages. The columns represent the number of observations performed (n = 176)

posed to patients' microphages, a high number of immigrating leukocytes was found (Fig. 3). Finally, microphages from volunteers incubated with autologous spermatozoa showed no chemotactic activity (Fig. 4). Statistical analysis demonstrated a significant increase of chemotactic activity against both autologous and homologous sperm for the microphages from patients when compared with the control ($P \leq 0.001$).

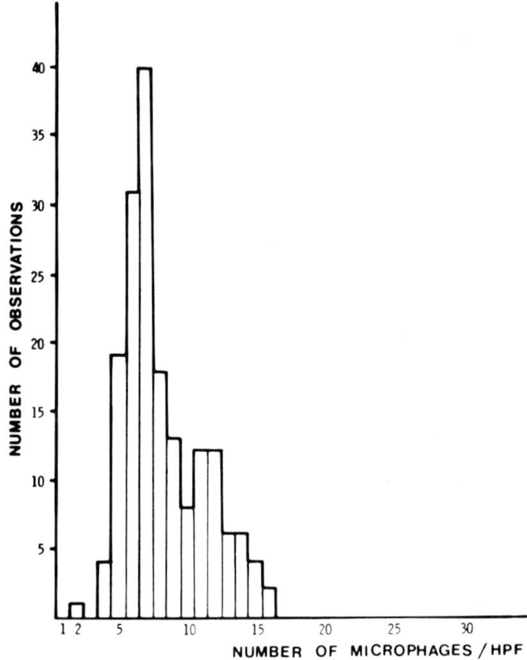

Fig. 2. Patients' spermatozoa incubated with microphages from volunteers. The columns represent the number of observations performed (n = 176)

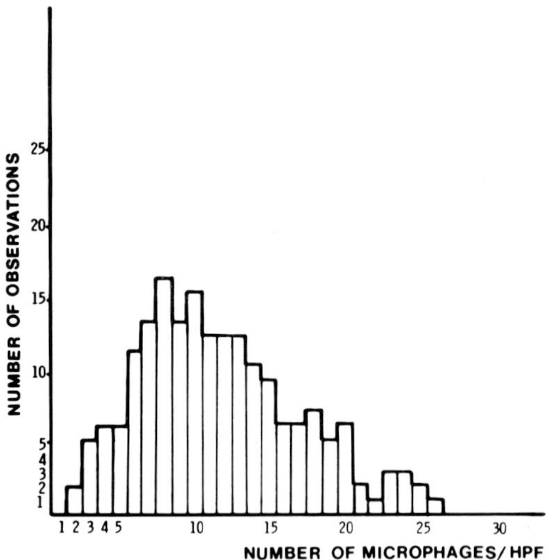

Fig. 3. Volunteers' spermatozoa incubated with microphages from patients. The columns represent the number of observations performed (n = 184)

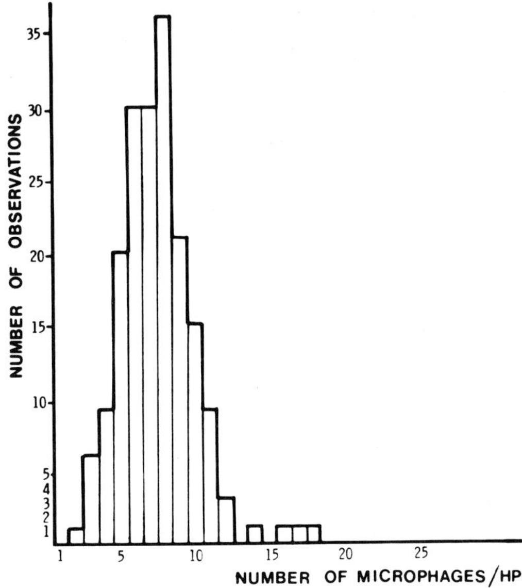

Fig. 4. Volunteers' spermatozoa incubated with autologous microphages. The columns represent the number of observations performed (n = 184)

This enhanced antispermatozoan activity of microphages from patients with a varicocele might resemble a nonimmunologic reaction for removal of debris. It might, however, indicate the development of a specific autoimmunologic process influencing and possibly reducing fertility [4, 5].

References

1. Djawari D, Bischoff Th, Hornstein OP (1978) Impairment of chemotactic activity of microphages in chronic mucocutaneous candidosis. Arch Dermatol Res 262:247–253
2. Jecht E (1977) Zur Pathogenese der Varikozelen-bedingten Fertilitätsstörungen. In: Semm K, Rauscher H, Schirren C (eds) Fortschritte der Fertilitätsforschung V. Grosse, Berlin, p 80
3. Jecht E (1979) Fertilitätsstörungen des Mannes. Moderne Medizin 7:1382–1387
4. Maroni ES, Wilkinson PC (1971) Selective chemotaxis of macrophages toward human and guinea-pig spermatozoa. J Reprod Fertil 27:149–152
5. Phadke AM (1975) Spermiophage cells in man. Fertil Steril 26:760–774

V. Therapy

A. Surgical Treatment

Surgical Treatment of Varicocele

K. M. Schrott

Surgical interventions on varicocele (e.g., local resection of the venous pampiniform plexus with and without orchipexy, internal suspension of testis with and without venectomy, shrinking of testis by plastic operation, bloody varicosclerosation) often yield unsatisfactory results. Frequently occurring recidivations, venous stases, neuralgias of the spermatic cord, orchiatrophies, and thromboses justify the demand for an exact indication for surgery and often also for its refusal.

Modified Indication for Surgery

Suprainguinal ligation of the internal spermatic vessels, which is increasingly becoming the method of choice [1, 8], has fundamentally changed the indication for surgery on varicocele. As this method is technically simple, without risk to the patient, and of therapeutic effectiveness, we can recommend this for a wide range of indications today. An operation is indicated whenever a patients feels troubled by a varicocele. This is not only when definite local evidence of a varicocele occurs with static or organic complaints or at the beginning of orchiatrophy but also with subfertility and infertility, which can be often found in such patients. Their treatment is the most important indication for surgery. Andrologists require the suprainguinal ligature to be carried out even in cases of subfertility alone with a typical pathologic spermiogram [2, 3, 7].

Because of their insignificant and temporary effect, conservative measures, such as the formerly practised cold water ablutions or suspensorys, should be abandoned in favor of the suprainguinal ligature.

Operative Technique

Today, the suprainguinal ligation of the internal spermatic vein [1, 5] is the method of choice in the operative treatment of a primary varicocele, as demonstrated by anatomical and phlebographic studies [4] while the intrainguinal approach bears more risks [6]. The operation technique is simple, safe, and riskless. A gridiron incision (Fig. 1) is made about 2–3 cm above the inner inguinal ring parallel to the inguinal ligament. After distraction of the musculature, we find the internal spermatic vessels adherent to the peritoneum. They can easily be found when the patient lies in an oblique position, thus avoiding a collapse of the internal spermatic veins.

Fig. 1. Access with gridiron incision
for suprainguinal ligature of the
internal spermatic vein

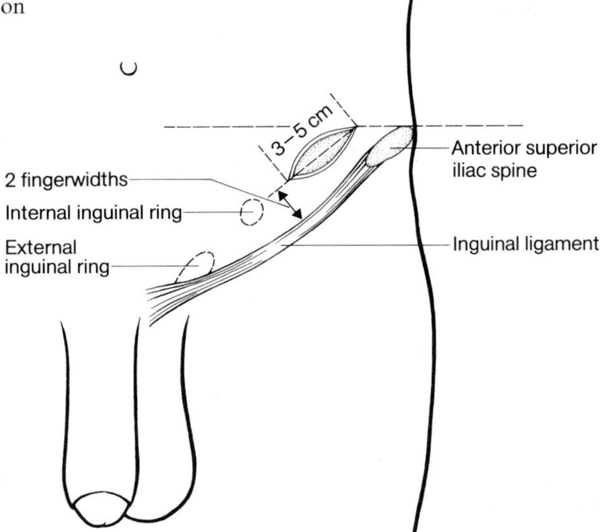

After the relatively delicate internal spermatic artery has been loosened, the veins, which are often arranged in pairs, can be ligated and transected to cranial and caudal. This procedure has the great advantage that venous anastomoses between the deep and superficial venous system of testis and epididymis remain uninjured. Not only does the internal spermatic artery remain intact but also the entire arterial supply via the deferential and the external spermatic artery.

In the case of an unclear anatomic situation, the surgeon should look for the branch of the deferent duct; the ligature of the vein must always be carried out cranially from it.

Ligation of the Internal Spermatic Artery

The same operation success can be obtained if the internal spermatic artery [8] is ligated in addition to the internal spermatic vein. Today, it is known that orchiatrophy will not occur if both the external spermatic artery and the deferential artery are intact. There, however, lies the decisive disadvantage of this method, for it is contraindicated at all primary operations in the pelvic ureteral section or in that of the inguinal channel, the testis, and the scrotum, whereas no contraindication is known for the ligation of the spermatic vein alone.

Results

The operation results of both methods are equally impressive. The suprainguinal ligature relieves the hydrostatic pressure so that the veins of the pampiniform plexus can collapse. For a few days, a transient insignificant edema may develop in the scrotal skin. A suspensory is recommended for 2 weeks.

In general the cosmetic effect is very good, because the elongation of the scrotum recedes. Subjective complaints nearly always disappear.

Complications such as recidivation, orchiatrophies, neuralgias of the spermatic cord, thromboses in the pampiniform plexus, or other complications are unknown with this method.

The functional results are likewise impressive. A comparison of the spermiogram before and 1 year after the suprainguinal ligature generally shows that the sperm count has doubled. The more distinctive the preoperative oligospermia, the higher is the relative increase of the cell number. A sperm count of 20–40 million per milliliter is considered to be sufficient.

Only 5% of the patients with varicocele who undergo an operation have a sufficient sperm motility index. After surgery, however, an improved motility with a sufficient activity index of 40%–50% of motile cells can be found in more than 60% of the patients.

About 90% of the patients with varicocele have less than 60% of normal spermatozoas in the preoperative spermiogram as against a normal rate of more than 80%. In these cases, too, a significantly improved spermatogenesis is obvious and about 40% of the operated patients are potent 1 year later [3, 9].

References

1. Bernardi R (1942) New incision for therapy of varicocele; semeiologic and surgical concepts. Sem Med 2:165 and Bol Inst Clin Quir (B. Aires) 18:323
2. Brown JS, Dubin L, Becker M, Hotchkiss RS (1967) Venography in the subfertile man with varicocele. J Urol 98:388
3. Campbell MF, Harrison JH (1970) Urology vol I. Saunders, Philadelphia, pp 173–174, 621–624, 674–682
4. Gösfay S (1959) Untersuchungen der Vena spermatica interna durch retrograde Phlebographie bei Kranken mit Varicocele. Z Urol 52:105
5. Hegemann G, Schmitz W (1968) Die suprainguinale Gefäßresektion bei Varicocelen aus chirurgisch-anatomischer Sicht. Z Urol 61:3
6. Ivanissevich O (1924) Las venas espermaticas del lado izquierdo. Estado en 40 desecciones cadavericas y en 20 operaciones por hernia y varicocele. Sem Med 1:1191
7. McLeod J (1965) Seminal cytology in the presence of varicocele. Fertil Steril 16:735
8. Palomo A (1949) Radical cure of varicocele by a new technique: Preliminary report. J Urol 61:604
9. Scott LS, Young D (1962) Varicocele: A study of its effects on human spermatogenesis, and of the results produced by spermatic vein ligation. Fertil Steril 13:47

Recidivation of Varicocele, Prophylaxis, and Therapy

D. Völter and A. J. Keller

The operation method preferred in therapy of idiopathic varicocele in recent years is increasingly the suprainguinal ligature of the v. testicularis, as described first by Bernardi in 1941. Postoperatively, a recidivation of the varicocele or a persistent varicocele can be expected in more than 10% of all cases. The reason for a persistent varicocele in more than 90% of all cases is an incomplete ligature of the branches of the V. testicularis. To reduce this high rate of failure some authors principally demand phlebography before every operation of varicocele [2]. It is questionable, however, if this step can achieve a reasonable reduction of the failure rate, because in phlebography smaller branches of the v. testicularis responsible for the persistence of varicocele cannot be shown in all cases. A much safer method to reduce the high failure rate of more than 10% is to ligate the vasa testiculares completely. This operation method, which was first described by Palomo [8] in 1949, in our opinion, has been wrongly brought into discredit. It is true that an additional ligature of the a. testicularis is not necessary for a good postoperative result [3]. In most cases, however, ligation of the whole vascular bundle of the a. and v. testicularis can prevent the recidivation or persistence of the varicocele after high ligation of the v. testicularis. This can be concluded from the fact that the v. testicularis in 70% of patients consists of two or three veins above the inner inguinal ring [12]. Additionally, in 30% of cases the v. testicularis has a double, in 3% of cases a triple, orifice at the left v. renalis [12].

Preoperative vasography of a simple varicocele is, in our minds, an unreasonable demand on the patient [5]. This measure cannot prevent recidivation of the varicocele, because with scrotal as well as with transfemoral phlebography, the branches of the v. testicularis can be figured incompletely or not at all [13]. The latter is supported by Marberger, who reported a widened vessel which he saw in phlebography. After the ligature of this vessel in control phlebography of the still-persisting varicocele, a completely different vein appeared, which was not represented at the first examination [7]. Obviously after transfemoral as well as after scrotal phlebography, only the region of the main flow can be figured. If these smaller branches of the v. testicularis not represented in phlebography are not tied up during the operation, relapse of the varicocele can be expected. High ligature of the whole bundle of the vasa testiculares after Palomo prevents the surgeon from overlooking a small branch of the vein especially in stout patients. It has not been proved so far whether simultaneous ligation of the a. testicularis has disadvantageous consequences.

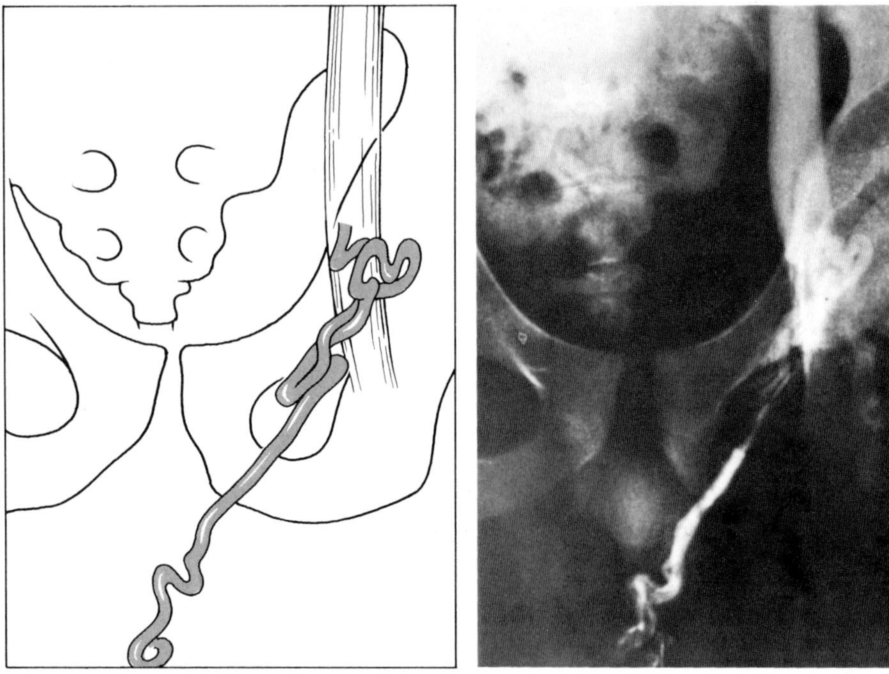

Fig. 1 a, b. Phlebography of a vein of the plexus pampiniformis. The contrast fluid flows exclusively through the v. iliaca externa

Follow-up examinations after high ligation of the v. testiculares in the Palomo method show an improvement of spermiogenesis in two-thirds of the patients just as after the isolated ligature of only the v. testicularis in the Bernardi method [6].

To date, only experiments with rabbits are known, in which the simultaneous ligation of the a. testicularis can cause changes of the testicular epithelium [1]. The results of these animal experiments, however, allow no statement about the conditions in man.

In most of the patients with persistent varicocele, phlebography shows one or several unligated branches of the testicular vein.

In some patients, however, phlebography shows that the main blood flow is from the plexus pampiniformis, which means most of the retrograde stream of blood is not running through the v. testicularis. In these patients the flow is drained into the v. iliaca externa, possibly via the v. spermatica externa which drains into the v. epigastrica inferior (Fig. 1). In the case of this anomaly, we prefer as the second operation method the evacuation of the spermatic cord below the musculus rectus abdominis according to Giuliani [4].

For the evacuation of the funiculus according to Giuliani, an inguinal incision and the opening of the inguinal canal is necessary. After luxation of the testis (Fig. 2) the fascia m. recti is incised in the linea alba. Now the testis can be pulled through the preperitoneal under the musculus rectus abdominis (Fig. 3). The spermatic cord finally lies under the musculus rectus abdominis. After this the inguinal

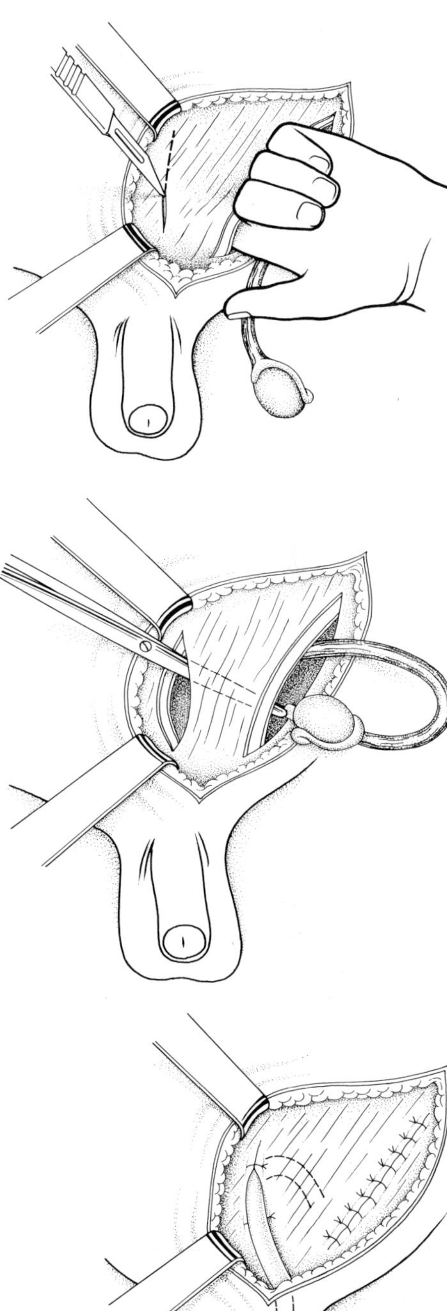

Fig. 2. After luxation of the testis out of the scrotum, the rectus fascia is incised above the preperitoneal lying finger. Reprinted from [9]

Fig. 3. With a forceps, the testis is pulled through preperitoneal below the m. rectus abdominis. Reprinted from [9]

Fig. 4. The spermatic cord lies below the m. rectus abdominis. The inguinal canal is closed according to the Bassini method. Reprinted from [9]

canal is closed according to Bassini (Fig. 4) and the testis transferred back into the scrotum. Because of this lengthening of the funiculus, a compression of widened veins can be obtained. Thus, in more than 70% of the cases a substantial improvement of the spermiogramm can be achieved [11].

We conclude with the following points:

1. The best prophylaxis against recidivation of varicocele is the high ligation of the vasa testiculares according to the Palomo method. Only in this way can the ligature of even very small branches of the v. testicularis be obtained with safety.
2. Some years ago, high ligation of the vasa testicularia according to Palomo was discontinued, although poor results of postoperative spermatogenesis were not reported. Control examinations of spermiograms in extensive alternate rows are completely lacking. Results after high ligature of the v. testiculares according to Palomo and results after isolated ligature of the v. testicularis according to Bernardi should be compared.
3. In preoperative phlebography, which should not be carried out in the case of simple varicocele, small vein branches of v. testicularis are generally not filled by contrast medium and not seen.

Only in very rare cases, such as when the main blood flow of the plexus pampiniformis does not run through the v. testicularis, is routine phlebography able to prevent the need for a second operation. In our opinion these patients should be operated upon a second time, shifting the spermatic cord under the musculus rectus abdominis according to Giuliani [10].

References

1. Baumgärtel H, Riedel B (1971) Die Durchblutung des Kaninchenhodens nach Ligatur der Vasa spermatica interna. Verh Dtsch Ges Urol 23:262
2. Egger B, Forster D, Mauermayer W, Sedlmayer G (1979) Die präoperative Phlebographie der Vena spermatica bei Rezidivoperationen der Varikozele. In: Weber W, Jonas D, Reinterventionen an den Urogenitalorganen. Thieme, Stuttgart, pp 274
3. Gasser G, Mayer HG (1977) Varikozele. Verh Dtsch Ges Urol 28:442
4. Giuliani GM (1955) Trasposizione del cordone o funicolo spermatico nel trattamento chirurgico del varicocele nell'uomo. Arch Ital Chir 80:51
5. Klosterhalfen H, Schirren C, Wagenknecht LV (1979) Pathogenese und Therapie der Varicocele. Urologe [A] 18:187
6. Kolle P, Vogel PG, Fuchs R (1971) Indikation und Ergebnisse der hohen Ligatur der spermatischen Gefäße nach Palomo. Verh Dtsch Ges Urol 23:250
7. Marberger H (1977) Diskussionsbemerkung. Verh Dtsch Ges Urol 28:340
8. Palomo A (1949) Radical cure of varicocele by a new technique. J Urol 61:604
9. Staehler W, Völter D (1977) Die Operationen an den männlichen Geschlechtsorganen. In: Bier, Braun, Kümmel (eds) Chirurgische Operationslehre, 8. Aufl. Barth, Leipzig, pp 429
10. Völter D, Feneis H (1978) Das Varikozelenrezidiv. Urologe [A] 17:242
11. Völter D, Lüders G, Oswald K (1971) Indikation und vergleichende Ergebnisse der Varicocelenoperation nach Giuliani und Palomo. Verh Dtsch Ges Urol 23:257
12. Völter D, Wurster J, Aeikens B, Schubert GE (1975) Untersuchungen zur Struktur und Funktion der Vena spermatica interna. Andrologia 7:127
13. Weißbach L, Janson R (1979) Die transfemorale Phlebographie der Vena testicularis vor der Operation des sog. Varikozelen-Rezidivs. In: Weber W, Jonas D, Reinterventionen an den Urogenitalorganen. Thieme, Stuttgart, pp 280

Persisting Varicocele: Cause and Treatment

L.V. WAGENKNECHT, R. HUBMANN, C. SCHIRREN, and H. VOGEL

Varicocele is one of the most frequent causes of male subfertility and has enormous practical importance because it can be treated surgically [1–3]. Varicocele was found in 17% of 3 million recruitment examinations in Germany. Studies by American investigators could demonstrate a varicocele in more than 20% of an unselected population and in up to 39% of infertility patients [8]. According to Schirren and Klosterhalfen, 40% to 50% of the patients with varicocele suffer from oligo-zoospermia.

Patients Material

During the past 16 years, 631 patients have undergone varicocele operations in the Department of Urology, University of Hamburg.

Follow-up controls in 287 patients demonstrated an improved spermiogram in 240 patients, and 58 patients of the latter informed us of a pregnancy.

Because of persisting varicocele, five of our patients, as well as 13 patients operated upon before in other clinics required a second operation.

Normal Venous Anatomy

The venous blood of the testis and epididymis is collected in the pampiniform plexus and drains off in three different ways: through the testicular vein (internal spermatic vein); through the cremasteric vein (external spermatic vein); and through the deferential vein.

The cremasteric vein drains into the epigastric vein, a satellite vein to the external iliac vein. The deferential vein, however, drains into the superior vesical vein and the internal iliac vein. At the level of the external inguinal ring, anastomoses exist with the pudendal and epigastric veins. The testicular vein, which is important for the pathogenesis of varicoceles, develops from a subcardinal vein. It opens on the left side into the renal vein and on the right side into the caval vein [1, 3–5, 7], nearly always at an right angle about 4 cm below the orifice of the renal vein.

Radiologic Visualization

Retrograde demonstration of the testicular vein is a quick and easy procedure. After puncture of the right femoral vein, a preshaped catheter is advanced through the renal vein into the testicular vein (Fig. 1). The latter usually opens into the renal vein about 6 cm laterally toward the lower border of the opening of the renal vein into the inferior caval vein [7]. Normally, this conforms with the lower renal vein contour. Venous valves, if present, are near the orifice. In its course, the vein crosses with the ureter. Sometimes the crossing point is marked on the ureter by a small crena. The catheter can be advanced caudally over a guide wire. Five minutes after puncture of the femoral vein the catheter is placed in its proper position in most cases. Subsequently, contrast material can be injected either by hand or mechanically under low pressure.

If distal anatomic conditions are to be examined, the pictures must be made with a sheet-film changer with the patient in a supine position. Visualization of a varicocele, however, should be performed with the patient in an oblique position on a tilting table [1]. If, in special cases, an orifice into the renal vein cannot be found, phlebography of the renal vein with a balloon catheter should be performed.

Visualization by contrast material injection after exposure of the deep veins of the pampiniform plexus at the root of the scrotum or of the testicular vein in the inguinal canal does not appear easier in comparison to the procedure described above (Fig. 2).

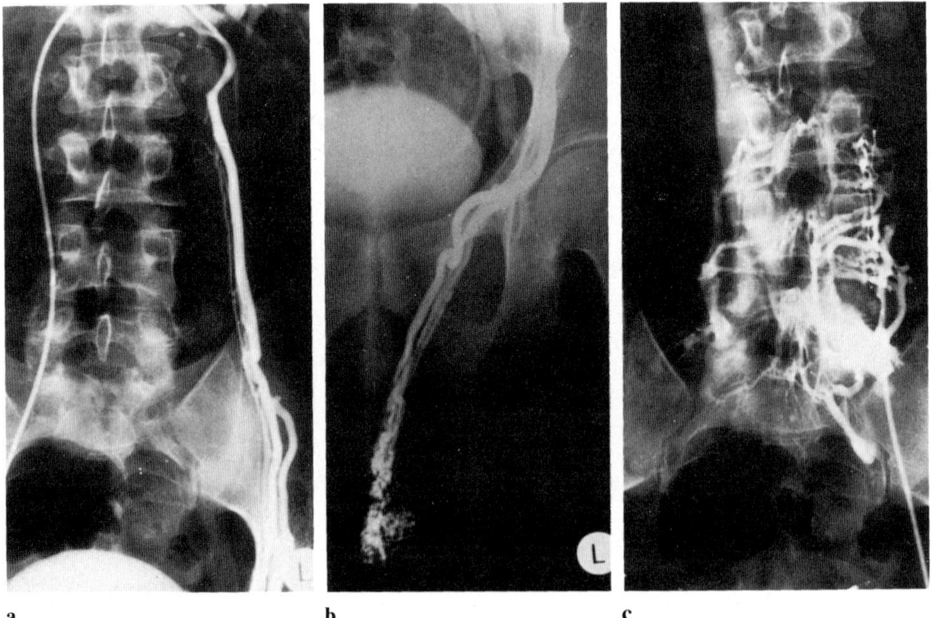

a   b   c

Fig. 1a–c. Preoperative phlebography of the internal spermatic vein in varicoceles. **a** Super-selectively catheterized internal spermatic vein with branches. **b** Varicocele. **c** Retrograde phlebography of the paravertebral plexus

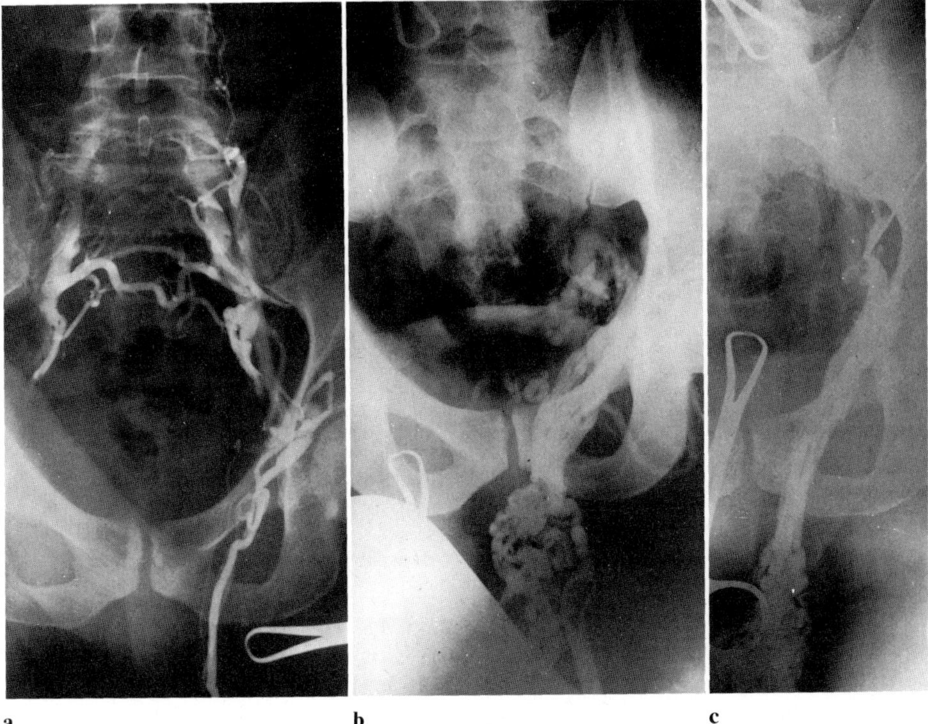

Fig. 2a–c. Intraoperative phlebography. **a** Venous anastomoses with the iliac vein, the paravertebral plexus, and presacral to the other side. **b** Collateral veins to the femoral vein, parasacral, and via the pampiniform plexus to the other side. **c** Venous drainage through collaterals to the iliac vein (proved by operation)

Causes of Failure of Preoperative Phlebography

Numerous anatomic variations are known. Some of them may be responsible for unsuccessful attempts to carry out an angiography and are therefore worth mentioning:

1. The left renal vein may be arranged like a circumaortal ring. If the probing of one side of this ring is unsuccessful, one should look for the orifice of the testicular vein on the other side.
2. Anastomoses with the system of the ascendent lumbar vein frequently occur. The contrast material, if injected into the distal section, may flow off through these anastomoses, thus impeding a visualization of the proximal vascular section. In this case, one should make an attempt to advance the catheter proximally beyond the anastomosis.
3. A direct communication of the renal vein with the ascendent lumbar vein can be mistaken for the testicular vein. Such atypical communication, however, is always located more medially [5]. The main reason for unsuccessful attempts are venous valves which cannot be passed by the catheter.

4. In the case of persisting varicocele, a superselective demonstration of the paravertebral plexus (Fig. 1 c) sometimes proves necessary to visualize collaterals of
   the internal spermatic vein.

Persisting Varicocele

During the past 16 years, 18 patients have undergone second operations in this hospital because of postoperatively persisting varicocele. A persistency of varicocele
(Fig. 3) after two operations is a rarity. We saw three such cases.

The most frequent cause of a persisting varicocele is a branch of the internal
spermatic vein overlooked in the first operation and later dilated (Table 1, Fig. 4).
Sometimes, this branch may be located extremely medially and, in the adherent
peritoneum, defy visualization and ligation.

Occasionally, a loosened ligation of the internal spermatic vein can be observed
and demonstrated by phlebography.

Intraoperative phlebography (Fig. 4) can reveal additional anastomoses, e.g., with
the paravertebral or presacral plexus, the femoral vein, the iliac vein, and to the
other side via the pampiniform plexus. However, a longer incision was necessary in
three cases for the ligation of the discovered collaterals.

For better planning of the operation, we therefore prefer the relatively easy procedure of *preoperative phlebography.* In single cases, only the selective demonstration of the prevertebral plexus will discover functional collaterals or preclude
them with certainty (Fig. 1 c).

We have demonstrated the superiority of preoperative phlebography in a comparative study in 13 patients with persisting varicocele. Figure 4 shows on the left,
preoperative phlebography and, on the right, the difficult and incomplete intraoperative phlebography.

Previously undiscovered anastomoses of the internal spermatic vein (Fig. 5) with
the paravertebral and presacral venous network were found, presacrally to the other
side to renal capsular veins to the femoral, and to the iliac vein as well as via the
pampiniform plexus to the other side.

In the case of bilaterally persisting varicocele we found three overlooked
branches as well as lateral and paravertebral ramifications.

Table 1. Causes of Persisting Varicocele

Result of phlebography		No. of cases
Overlooked branch of the int.sperm.v.		2
Collaterals to paravertebral plexus		3
Overlooked branches and collaterals		13
collateral veins to iliac vein	7	
anastomoses with femoral vein	6	
collateral veins to other side (pampiniform plexus)	2	
presacral and paravertebral collaterals	9	
Total		18

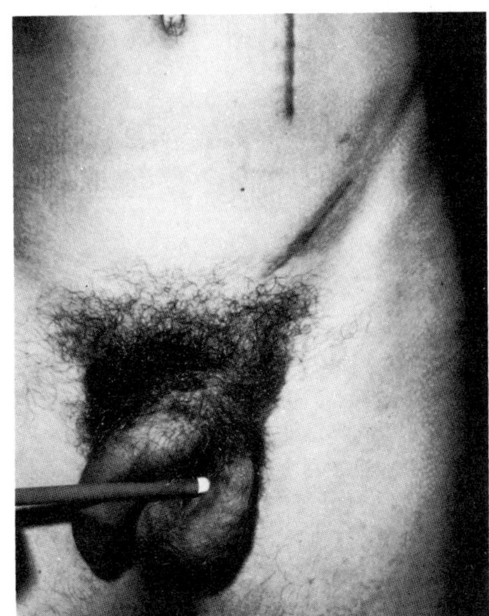

Fig. 3. Persisting varicocele after two operations

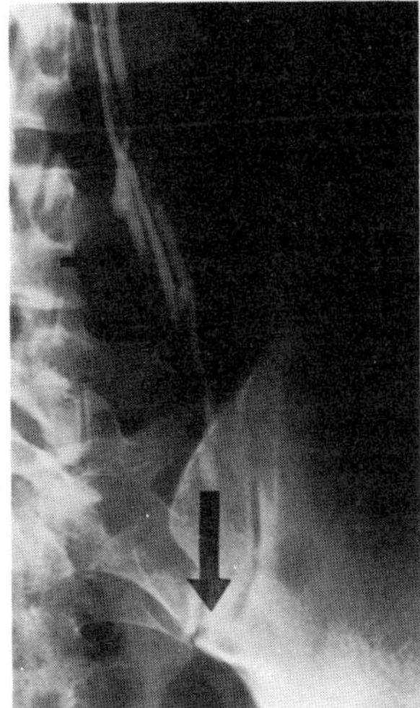

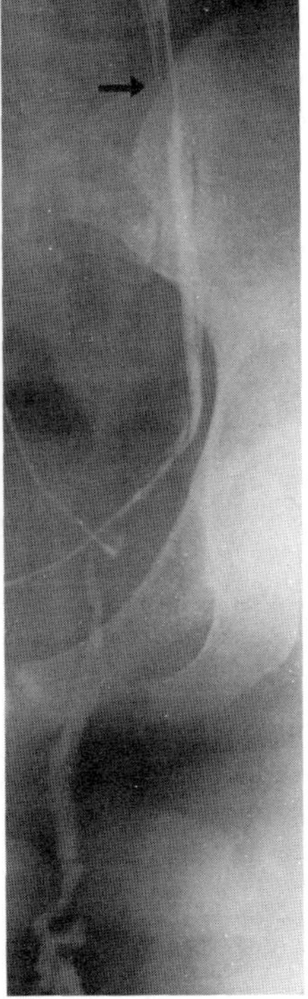

Fig. 4. Comparison of preoperative *(left)* and intraoperative *(right)* phlebography. (Small arrows: ligated trunks of testicular vein, large arrow: unligated – persistent – trunk of testicular vein)

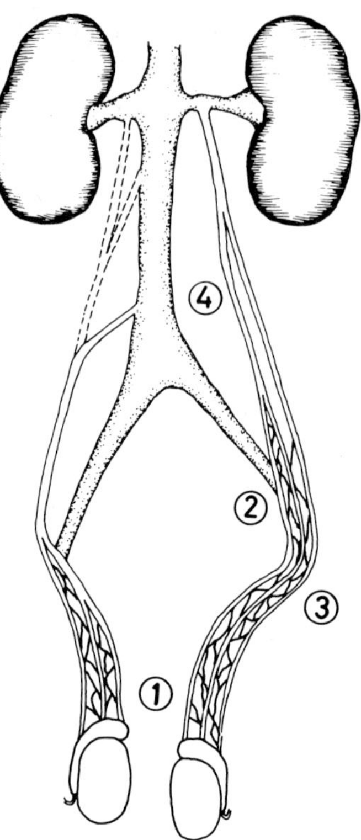

Fig. 5. Various collateral veins of the internal spermatic vein in persisting varicocele: (1) via the pampiniform plexus to the other side; (2) to the iliac vein; (3) to the femoral vein; and (4) to the presacral and paravertebral plexus

In 17 patients a second operation was necessary because of varicocele on the left side, in one patient on both sides. In 2 cases the cause was solely an overlooked branch; in 3 cases, an anastomosis with the paravertebral plexus; and in 13 cases, other collaterals (Table 1).

Table 2 could convey the impression that high ligation has the highest persistency rate. However, it should be taken into account that this operation is the most common one; a valid comparison of the different techniques is not yet available.

Table 2. Surgical Techniques for Persisting Varicocele

Operation	No. of cases		
	1st op.	2nd. op.	3rd op.
Bernardi technique (pararectal mesogastric incision)	11	4	
Ivanissevich technique (pararectal hypogastric incision)	3	3	3
Palomo technique (inguinal incision)	4	11	
Total	18	18	3

In our opinion, the surgical technique proposed by Palomo is illogical, since the additional ligation of the testicular artery cannot improve an already impaired spermiogram.

Conclusion

Ligation of the internal spermatic vein in cases of varicocele and subfertility is the most successful single therapeutic procedure practised in andrologic urology. For high ligation, pararectal incision is recommended because of the venous ramification which increases caudally.

In our material of more than 600 patients operated upon in this way, the failure rate was 1%[1]. Causes that made a second operation necessary were overlooked branches and undiscovered collaterals to neighboring venous systems.

Preoperative phlebography is the method of choice for visualization of such anomalies in order to allow optimal preoperative planning.

Abstract

We report on 18 patients presenting persisting varicoceles following one or several surgical attempts to ligate the internal spermatic vein. In this center during the last 16 years, 631 patients underwent high ligation of the internal spermatic vein (technique of Bernardi) for varicocele. In five of them varicocele persisted after surgery (1%).

Phlebography in the 18 cases operated upon showed: an overlooked branch of the internal spermatic vein in two cases; collateral veins to the paravertebral plexus in three cases; and a combination of venous collaterals to neighboring systems with overlooked branches in 13 cases. Collateral anastomoses as a cause for persisting varicoceles were demonstrated connecting to the presacral- and paravertebral plexus, and to the iliac vein and the femoral vein to renal capsular veins and via the pampiniform plexus to the other side. Preoperative phlebography is preferred to intraoperative radiological examination since the latter may be technically difficult, incomplete, and may require a longer incision for ligation of distant anastomoses.

References

1. Ahlberg NE, Bartley O, Chikedel N, Fritjofsson A (1966) Phlebography in varicocele scroti. Acta Radiol [Diagn] 4:517
2. Bandhauer K, Meili HM (1977) Varicocele, Spermiogramm, Hodenbiopsie – Plasmatestosteron – Therapieergebnisse. Urologe [A] 16:154
3. Frick J, Bantlow K (1969) Die Angiografie der li. V. spermatica. ROEFO 111:241
4. Gösfay S (1959) Untersuchungen der V. spermatica interna durch retrograde Phlebografie bei Kranken mit Varicocele. Z Urol 52:105

---

1 Editors' note: 287 patients were followed-up of whom 5 required a second operation (cf. patient material. Also, cf. page 173).

5. Jacobs JB (1969) Selective gonadal venography. Radiology 92:885
6. Klosterhalfen H, Wagenknecht LV, Schirren C (to be published) Pathogenese and Therapie der Varicocele. Urologe [A]
7. Lien HH, Kolbenstvedt A (1977) Phlebographic appearances of the left renal and left testicular veins. Acta Radiol [Diagn] 18:321
8. Verstoppen GR, Steeno OP (1977, 1978) Varicocele and the pathogenesis of the associated subfertility. A review of the various theories. Part I: Andrologie 9:133; Part II: Andrologie 9:293; Part III: Andrologie 10:85
9. Völter D, Feneis H (1978) Das Varicocelenrezidiv. Urologe [A] 17:242–244
10. Wagenknecht LV, Hubmann R, Schirren C, Erbe W (to be published) Ursachen der postoperativ fortbestehenden Varicocele. Andrologie
11. Weißbach L, Janson R (1979) Die transfemorale Phlebografie der Vena testicularis vor der Operation des. sog. Varicocelenrezidivs. In: Reinterventionen an den Urogenitalorganen, Weber W, Jonas D (eds) Thieme, Stuttgart, p 280

B. Sclerotherapy

Results of Transfemoral Testicular Vein Obliteration Using a Balloon Catheter

P. RIEDL and G. LUNGLMAYR

In this symposium different techniques for transfemoral obliteration of the testicular vein are reviewed. At the University of Vienna Medical School, a coaxial catheter-balloon catheter system has been used for sclerosing in order to minimize the risk of sclerosant reflux into the renal vein [8, 9]. The technique has been routinely employed for the past 18 months in a total of 58 cases.

Material and Method

Patients were aged between 13 and 48 years (mean age, 26.2 years). In about 50% (22 cases), testicular vein obliteration was done because patients had wanted to have children for 6 months to 13 years; in the remaining cases obliteration was indicated for other reasons (accidental detection of varicocele on general check-up, pains, or increasing size of varicocele).

Prior to obliteration, and 1 week and 1, 3, 6, and 12 months after treatment, clinical examination, contact thermography, and spermatologic analysis were performed. The technique for obliteration using the balloon catheter system has been reported elsewhere [8, 9].

Results

Of the 144 patients undergoing selective testicular vein phlebography, 71 were scheduled for obliteration, which was successful in 58 cases (81.7%). Failures were due to anatomical factors in nine cases and to other causes (e.g., collapse of patient, fluoroscopy time exceeding self-imposed limits) in four (Table 1).

Table 2 lists the results of post-treatment palpation and contact thermographies. In 48 cases (82.8%), varicoceles completely disappeared. Six of the 10 patients with persistent or only slightly smaller varicoceles underwent repeat phlebography and reobliteration (Table 3), with complete disappearance of the varicocele in three cases.

Of the 36 patients who underwent treatment more than 3 months ago, 20 had improved spermiograms; in 9 cases spermiograms were unchanged, and 7 cases were worse than before (Table 4). In 15 of the 22 patients who had wanted children, the post-treatment interval is now longer than 3 months, and the partners of four of these patients have meanwhile conceived.

Table 1. Patient material

Selective retrograde testicular vein phlebography	No. of patients	%
Obliteration scheduled in	71	100.0
Obliteration successful in	58	81.7
Obliteration failed in	13	18.3
Reasons for failure:		
Anatomical factors	9	12.7
Other factors (collapse, etc.)	4	5.6

Table 2. Results of contact thermography and clinical examination in 58 obliterated testicular veins

Varicocele	After 1st obliteration	
	No. of patients	%
Complete disappearance	48	82.8
Reduction in size	7	12.1 ⎱ 17.2
No change	3	5.1 ⎰
Total	58	100.0

Table 3. Scrotal temperatures in six patients twice undergoing testicular vein obliteration

Patient	Testicular vein diameter	Scrotal temperature over varicocele	
		1st obliteration	2nd obliteration
C.A.	8 mm ↑↑↑	↓ ↑↑	↓ ○
ST.A	10 mm ↑↑↑	↑↑↑	↑↑
H.P.	8 mm ↑↑	↑	○
L.W.	12 mm ↑↑↑	↑	↑
N.G.	8 mm ↑↑	↑↑	↑↑
S.E.	9 mm ↑↑↑	↑↑	○

Table 4. Spermiograms in 36 patients 3–18 months after testicular vein obliteration

	No. of patients	%
Improved	20	55.5
Unchanged	9	25.0
Deteriorated	7	19.5
Total	36	100.0

Table 5. Complications of testicular vein obliteration in 58 cases

		No. of patients	%
Pains		7	12.1
Perivascular infiltration		4	6.9
Collapse		3	5.2
Venous thrombosis in			
pampiniform plexus	> 3 ms	11	19.0
	< 3 ms	0	0.0
Mean fluoroscopy time			2′
Mean treatment time			16′
(from CM injection to obliteration)			

Transitory scrotal vein thrombosis was palpated in 11 instances, but disappeared in all cases within some months. Perivascular infiltration of the radiopaque substance in the area of the proximal testicular vein was found to be present in four cases; seven patients complained of transitory low-grade pain (Table 5). Serious complications of longer duration were absent.

Discussion

Transfemoral testicular vein obliteration using a balloon catheter is a novel technique for treatment of varicoceles. After 18 months' experience we feel justified in assessing the merits of the technique by comparing the results obtained with those of the established standard therapy, i.e., surgical ligation of the vein. Complications and success rates in terms of spermiogram quality and fertility are comparable with postoperative findings [5, 6. 14], while the rate of persisting varicoceles (10 of 58 cases, or 17.2%) is somewhat higher than after high suprainguinal ligation [1, 2, 4, 5, 7, 10, 14]. However, if veins with a diameter of more than 8 mm are excluded, the persistence rate is reduced to 3.5% (Tables 3 and 6).

While several novel alternatives for nonsurgical treatment of varicoceles are known, two factors argue in favor of transfemoral obliteration using the coaxial catheter-balloon-catheter technique. First, the action of the sclerosing agent is confined to the testicular vein, since the balloon catheter prevents reflux into the renal vein. Second, venous sclerosing agents have given excellent results for decades in the treatment of varices of the lower extremities [3, 11, 12, 13].

Table 6. Surgical ligation versus obliteration (sclerosing) of testicular vein

	Surgery	Obliteration
Improvement of spermiogram quality	60% – 80%	55%
Pregnancy	15% – 50%	25%
Complications	few	few
Persistence/relapse	1% – 20%	3.5% – 17%

Abstract

Fifty-eight patients with varicoceles underwent transfemoral obliteration of the testicular vein using a coaxial catheter-balloon catheter system. Treatment can be done on an outpatient basis and does not require anesthesia. Complications and success rates in terms of spermiogram quality and fertility are comparable with those of surgical treatment. Varicocele persistence appears to be more common than after surgical ligation.

References

1. Brown JS (1967) Varicocelectomy in the subfertile male: A ten-year experience with 295 cases. Fertil Steril 27:1046
2. Dubin L, Amelar RD (1975) Varicocelectomy as therapy in male infertility: A study of 504 cases. Fertil Steril 26:217
3. Feuerstein W, Mostbeck A (1977) Varizen-Verödung und Lungenembolierisiko. Phlebol Proktol 6:235
4. Fritjofsson A, Ahren C (1967) Studies on varicocele and subfertility. Scand J Urol Nephrol I:55
5. Greenberg SH (1977) Varicocele and male infertility. Fertil Steril 28:699
6. MacLeod J (1965) Seminal cytology in the presenca of varicocele. Fertil Steril 16:735
7. Mauss J, Schach H, Scheidt J (1974) Andrologische Untersuchungen bei subfertilen Männern vor und nach Carikocelenoperation. Hautarzt 25:394
8. Riedl P (1979) Selektive Phlebographie und Katheterthrombosierung der Vena testicularis bei primärer Varikocele. Wien Klin Wochenschr [Suppl] 91:99
9. Riedl P, Lunglmayr G, Stackl W (to be published) A new method of transfemoral testicular vein obliteration for varicocele using a ballon katheter. Radiology
10. Rost A, Richter-Reichhelm M, Kaden R, Pust R (1975) Die Varicocele als Ursache von Fertilitätsstörungen. Urologe [A] 14:282
11. Santler R, Kraft D (1975) Über Gerinnungsaktivitäten im Bereich der Venen. Phlebol Proktol 4:95
12. Sigg K (1976) Varizen, Ulcus cruris und Thrombose. Springer, Berlin Heidelberg New York
13. Steinacher J, Kammerhuber F (1968) Weg und Verweildauer eines Kontrastmittels im oberflächlichen Venensystem unter Bedingungen der Varizenverödung. Eine Studie zur Technik der Varizenverödung. Z Haut Geschlechtskr 43:369
14. Verstoppen GR, Steeno OP (1978) Varicocele and the pathogenesis of the associated subfertility. A review of the various theories. Andrologia 10:85

Sclerotherapy: Technique and Results

E. Zeitler, E.-I. Richter, W. Seyferth, and R. Grosse-Vorholt

The reports of Lima, Castro, and Costa [3], and Iaccarino [2] induced us to attempt occlusion therapy with a sclerosing agent by transfemoral phlebography of the internal spermatic vein in outpatients.

After consultation with colleagues particularly experienced in sclerotherapy [1], we decided to use Varicocid, as it is harmless and has a heavy sclerosing tendency. Varicocid is sodium morrhuate (55 mg) and benzyl alcohol (20 mg). Conditions for the application of the sclerosing agent are the selective catheterization of the internal spermatic vein and an evident opening insufficiency with a reflux longer than 5 cm of the contrast agent in the internal spermatic vein.

Sclerotherapy is aimed at the treatment of infertility and therefore is only justifiable in men of reproductive age. Varicocele in children, however, should be submitted to surgical treatment since the number, frequency, and extent of the recanalization after sclerotherapy is still unknown.

Sclerotherapy is carried out immediately upon phlebography proof of the varicocele.

The safe, specific location of the catheter in the internal spermatic vein is absolutely necessary for a sclerotherapeutic treatment. We use various catheter types with different bent tips and length of the flexed tip.

The opening of the internal spermatic vein varies in size, so for the catheterization of the left internal spermatic vein we either use home-made catheters with different curved tips or industrial-made (CORDIS) catheters, the last segment but one of them being 6 or 7 cm in length.

Because of difficult intubation into the internal spermatic vein, catheters with end or side holes are used occasionally for phlebography. Catheters without side holes are preferred for sclerotherapy.

Table 1. Methods of percutaneous treatment of varicoceles

I	II
Sclerotherapy with	Embolization with
A. Hypertonic glucose 75% + monoethanolamine	A. Gianturco technique
B. Varicocid	B. Detachable balloons
C. Aethoxysclerol	C. Bucrylate[a]

[a] Isobutyl 2-cyanoakrylate (IBC_2)

After phlebography, an examination is performed with the patient in a 30° upright oblique position in the X-ray apparatus. Besides optimal adjustment, temporary information, image documentation with fluorography, and Spot film technique 100×100 cm, special attention is paid to the radioprotection during fluoroscopy. The patient's testes are covered with a protective cap.

If the patient is in this position and does not have too wide an internal spermatic vein, and little or no contrast material entered the renal vein, we perform sclerotherapy with a phlebography catheter.

Whereas contrast media of low osmolality are used for diagnostic purposes, the ionic contrast medium Urografin 76% is used for therapeutic control, as a thrombosis-reducing effect of the contrast material is not desired.

A three-way cock is adapted to the end of the catheter through which first 1 ml of contrast medium is injected into the spermatic vein for marking the location of the sclerosing agent and then 3 ml Varicocid. The first injection is made under a slight Valsalva maneuver to allow the sclerosing agent to spread distally and to reach the collaterals or paired draining veins of the testes. After the injection of the sclerosing agent, another 1 ml of contrast medium is injected.

If, however, the lumen of the internal spermatic vein is so wide that an outflow of a large quantity of contrast medium into the renal vein can be prevented neither by an oblique positioning nor by a Valsalva maneuver, a balloon occlusion catheter is used. In this case the phlebography catheter is replaced over the guide wire by a catheter with a wide lumen (external diameter, 3.2 mm; internal diameter, 2.4 mm). Through this, a balloon catheter after Dotter[1] or Grünzig[3] is advanced into the spermatic vein. A slight injection of contrast medium inflates the balloon until contrast medium no longer flows through the main lumen into the renal vein. The sclerosing agent now can be applied with the patient slightly upright (30°) or in a horizontal position. A Valsalva maneuver is not required.

The coaxial catheter system with balloon was a time-consuming procedure and required additional screening time.

For this reason, we developed a double-lumen balloon catheter[2] for diagnostic and therapeutic treatment of the varicocele. The balloon is arranged 1 cm from the catheter tip and the Y-shaped connection allows separate injection of contrast material or sclerosing agent, or filling and draining of the balloon catheter. This or the Grüntzig double-lumen balloon catheter is of particular advantage for sclerotherapy, allowing both an optimal phlebography with the patient in a slightly upright position and sclerotherapy in every position, i.e., also with deep positioning of the head.

As the occluding catheter could relatively often be safely located in the internal spermatic vein, most of the sclerotherapeutic treatments were carried out on the left side. With growing experience, the percentage of successful catheterization of the right internal spermatic vein also increased. Both the catheter (306) normally used for the left side and the Sidewinder catheter 2 proved favorable for finding the right internal spermatic vein.

---

1 Cook Inc. Order No. TLV 4,8 French
2 Cordis S 393, 7 French
3 Schneider, Zürich, 6 mm, 3 cm

Only in the past 3 months, have we increasingly performed sclerotherapy on the right side, as we become more and more successful with the specific location of the catheter in the right internal spermatic vein and occlusion.

Decisive factors for a complete occlusion of the internal spermatic vein are as follows:

1. Safe, specific location of the catheter.

2. Local application of sclerosing agent. Upon safe local application, the majority of the patients feel an ache in the course of the internal spermatic vein which slowly diminishes after 1–2 min. If a complete occlusion cannot be achieved after the catheter or sclerosing agent has entered the renal vein through collaterals and cross connections, the patient notes a strange taste (violet-, almond-, or cod-liver oil-like). Consequently, a safe local application is not guaranteed, and special attention must be paid to an improved occlusion, a reinforced Valsalva maneuver or its omittance, and a modified positioning of the patient.

3. Duration of action of the sclerosing agent. After application of the sclerosing agent behind the occluding catheter, 10–15 min must elapse until the sclerosing effect develops and with it a local thrombosis. With a successful sclerotherapy, subsequent control phlebograms manifest an increasing reduction of the transverse lumen diameter of the internal spermatic vein and no diffusion of contrast agent distally. This means a complete occlusion with removal of the varicocele, or partial occlusion with transformation of a stage II or III varicocele into a stage I. These phases take place within an observation period of 10–30 min after application of sclerosing agent.
Following a control phlebography documenting the successful occlusion, the catheter is withdrawn from the spermatic vein into the renal vein and checked under fluoroscopic control to determine whether a Valsalva maneuver produces a reflux and whether the renal vein is patent.

The same procedure is to be applied for the right side. We have, however, less experience with the procedure on the right to date.

Table 2. Primary results of sclerotherapy in patients with varicocele (Aug. 1977–28 Feb. 1980)

Grades of internal spermatic vein insufficiency	Sclerotherapy		3 – 6 months later
	Before	After	
No spermatic v. insufficiency[a]	–	100	62
Grade I	4	16	3
Grade II	15	37	–
Grade III	136	2	–
n	155	155	65

[a] No varicocele

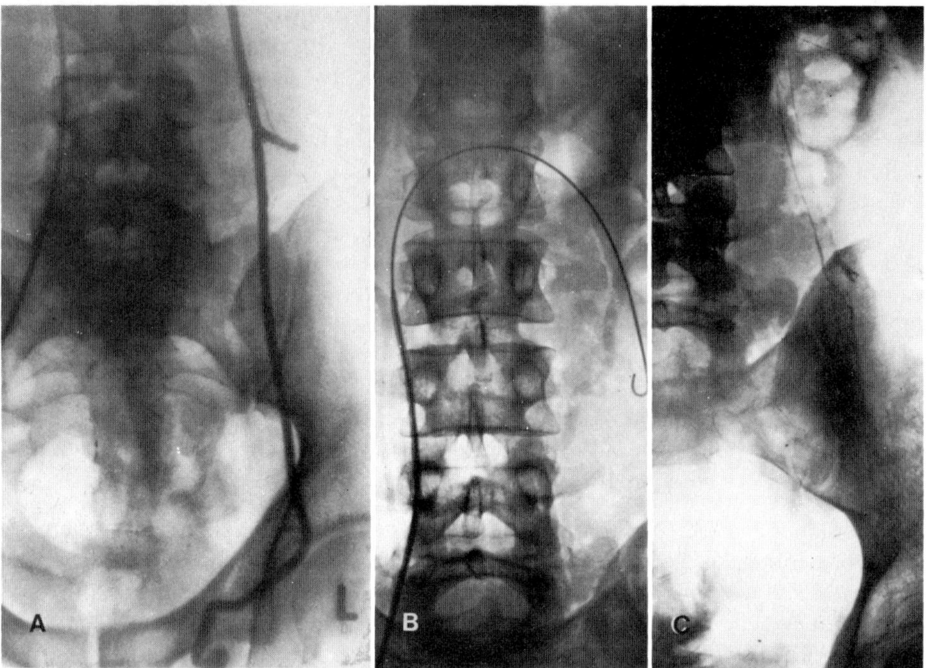

Fig. 1A–C. Left spermatic phlebography and sclerotherapy. **A** spermatic vein insufficiency stage III (with varicocele); **B** guide wire in the left spermatic vein; **C** situation after effective sclerotherapy

Of the 419 phlebographies of the internal spermatic vein we made (as of 29 February 1980), we found 287 varicoceles, stages I–III, on the left side. In 155 cases (53%), sclerotherapy was performed.

Special mention should be made that in the first 10 months, we carried out this examination procedure for diagnostic purposes only. Moreover, we desisted from sclerotherapy in all cases in which we suspected removal of a considerable quantity of sclerosing agent through the renal vein or its transport to other sections through cross connections. Above all, those cases were rejected in which the sclerosing agent was suspected to reach the paravertebral venous plexus. In all these cases we concluded the diagnostic procedure and recommended surgical intervention.

As we gained experience, the safe specific location of the catheter was also possible in the distal sections of the internal spermatic vein, and the number of varicoceles appropriate for undergoing sclerotherapy increased. As the success rate of selective catheterization of the right internal spermatic vein increased, sclerotherapy also increased on the right side. Twelve (21%) of the 57 varicoceles we proved on the right side were submitted to sclerotherapy up to 29 February 1980).

So far, however, the real share of right-sided varicoceles remains undecided.

Based on our recent experience, varicoceles on the right side might occur more often than so far suspected. Improvement of the diagnostic technique, however, might also lead to an improved therapeutic procedure for the right internal spermatic vein.

Fig. 2A–D. Phlebography with varicocele left and right. **A** spermatic vein insufficiency stage III (varicocele right); **B** spermatic vein insufficiency stage III (varicocele left)

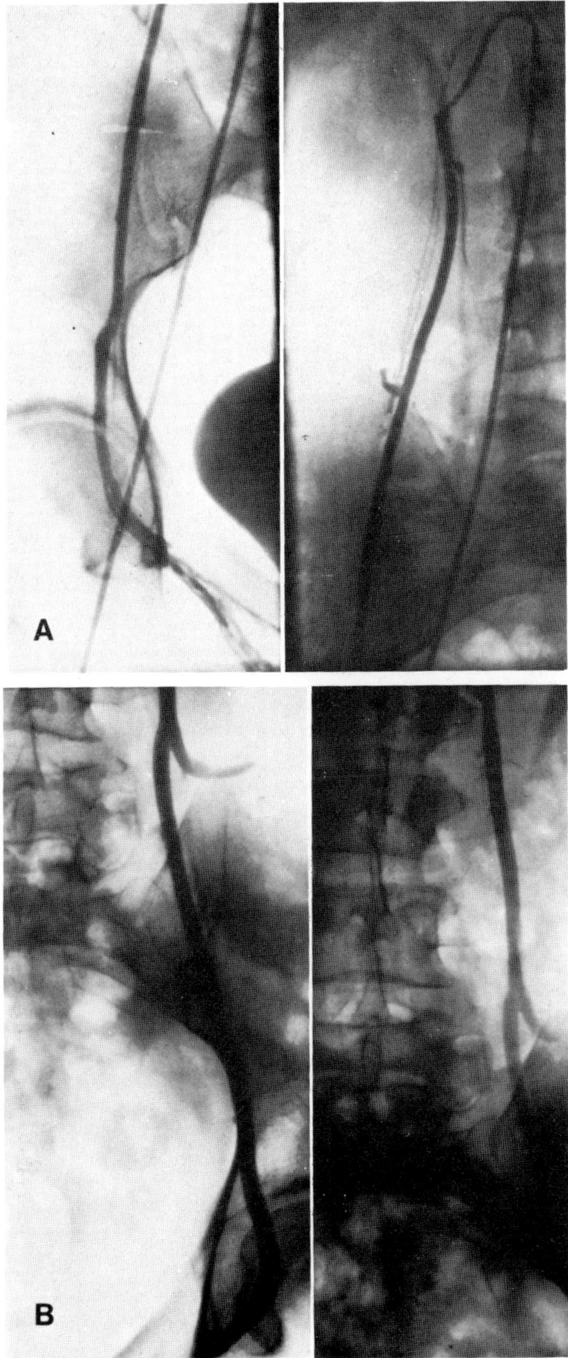

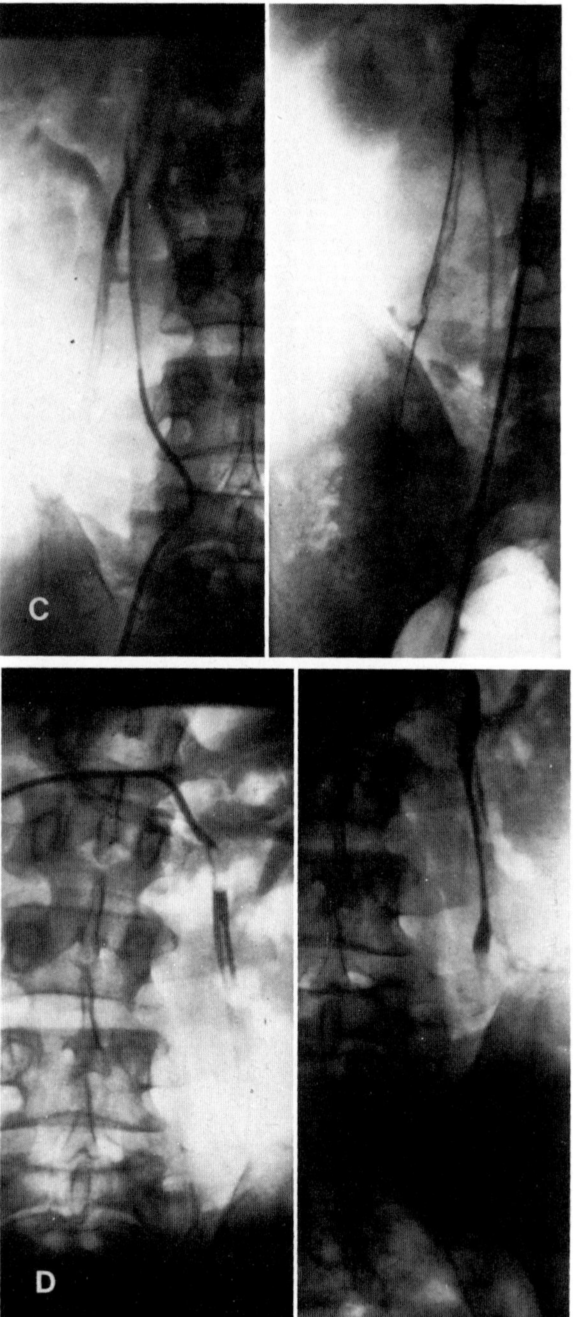

Fig. 2C u. D. Phlebography with varicocele left and right. **C** control phlebography with occluded spermatic vein after sclerotherapy (right); **D** control phlebography after sclerotherapy with occluded spermatic vein (left)

Results

In 164 left-sided varicoceles submitted to sclerotherapy so far, we were able to prove an occlusion only when performing the control phlebography 15 to 30 min after having applied the sclerosing agent. One to two ampoules of Varicocid were usually sufficient, and only in exceptional cases were up to five ampoules necessary. By that time the result was either the transformation of a stage II or III varicocele in a stage I, and frequently an occlusion up to 5 cm to the opening into the renal vein.

Follow-up controls 3–12 months later, made in 65 patients to date, manifested a complete occlusion in 62 cases (95%). This means that when making use of the diagnostic technique for phlebographic procedures, either a small proximal section only of the internal spermatic vein could be probed and no peripheral spreading of contrast material was provable during application, or a selective intubation was no longer possible. These findings indicate the desired occlusion, although selective intubation often fails at very narrow lumen.

Discussion

Bearing in mind the various treatment procedures, i.e., surgical ligature, local occlusion with metal coil spring or detachable balloon, and sclerotherapy, we decided to use sclerotherapy of the internal spermatic vein to treat varicoceles in patients with infertility for the following reasons:

1. Application of the sclerosing agent does not give rise to a local occlusion of the vein similar to the ligature, but causes an occlusion in the cross and longitudinal dimensions.
2. During the sclerosing procedure, even a large number of small distal and proximal connection veins which might give rise to recidivation are occluded.
3. Except for the very low risk of an idiosyncrasy sclerotherapy does not involve a real risk for the patient.

At present, we do not know exactly at what moment and to what extent recanalization sets in after sclerotherapy of the internal spermatic vein.

Conclusions analogous to the experiences obtained in peripheral veins can be made.

Even at recidivation after sclerotherapy or surgical treatment, sclerotherapy again can be performed if selective catheterization is possible. In 24 of 33 patients, postoperative control examinations revealed a persistent varicocele or recidivation. In 15 patients, a sclerotherapy was possible.

The results we have obtained so far show that, besides postoperative treatment, sclerotherapy of the internal spermatic vein in patients with varicocele is a method that offers good prospects for the treatment of the varicoceles, and with this of male infertility.

The clinical consequences of this technique will be reported in another article.

References

1. Haid-Fischer F, Haid H (1980) Venenerkrankungen. Phlebologie für Klinik und Praxis. 4. Aufl. Thieme, Stuttgart New York
2. Iaccarino V (1977) Trattamento conservativo del varicoseles: Flebografia selettiva o scleroterapia delle vene gonadiche. Riv Radiol 17:107–117
3. Lima SS, Castro MP, Costa OF (1978) A new method for the treatment of varicocele. Andrologia 10:103–106
4. Riedl P (1979) Varikozelen-Verödung. Muench Med Wochenschr 121:157
5. Riedl P (1979) Thrombosierung der Vena testicularis bei primärer Varikozele. Wien Klin Wochenschr (Suppl) 91:99
6. Zeitler E, Jecht E, Herzinger R, Richter E-I, Seyferth W, Grosse-Vorholt R (1979) Technik und Ergebnisse der Spermatika-Phlebographie bei 136 Männern mit primärer Sterilität. ROEFO 131:179–184
7. Zeitler E, Jecht E, Richter E-I, Seyferth W (1980) Perkutane Behandlung männlicher Infertilität im Rahmen der selektiven Spermatika-Phlebographie mit Katheter. ROEFO 132:293–300

C. Embolization

The Treatment of Idiopathic Varicocele by Transfemoral Spiral Occlusion of the Left Testicular Vein

M. Thelen, L. Weissbach, and P. Schramm

The increasingly frequent embolization therapy of arteries, the knowledge of the course of the testicular vein and its collaterals [7], as well as the development of embolization materials have given rise to the idea of introducing the embolization or sclerosing (Lima, Iaccarino, Zeitler) therapy of varicocele by venous occlusion as an alternative to surgical interventions. As for the available embolization materials, we think that the Gianturco spiral in addition to sclerosing agents [1, 3–6, 8] is appropiate for this new variant of transcutaneous catheter embolization.

Histoacryl, which might also have been used as an embolization material because of its adhesiveness, was discarded because it provokes extensive periadventitial inflammations, which may spread to the testicular artery, and sometimes the ureter. Moreover, it is not impossible that, in the long run, Histoacryl may provoke the appearance of granulomas or other reactions to foreign bodies. Other embolization materials could not be used because of the risk of dislocation and, consequently, embolization, of the pulmonary circulation via the renal vein.

Method

The spiral embolization of the testicular vein is preceded by diagnostic phlebography. The examination is done under local anesthesia; the starting point is the right groin. No concomitant medication is required. The catheter is introduced into the left renal vein, via the inferior vena cava, with the Seldinger technique. Then the reflux into the pampiniform plexus is proved and documented[1]; during this procedure, the patient should be in a 45° upright position and a Valsalva maneuver is carried out. The existence of the craniocaudal contrast blood stream is proof of pathologic hemodynamics of the insufficient venous system. The testicular vein is probed selectively; another injection of contrast medium serves to demonstrate the existence of collateral circulations.

The application of the embolization spiral depends on the existence of a venous insufficiency and the various courses of the vessels. The blocking-up serves either for the occlusion of a central vessel (Fig. 1) to which the said collaterals are tributaries, or for that of all collaterals; otherwise, the central trunk of a testicular vein, which ramifies towards the renal vein, has to be embolized.

---

1 We used Meglumin-Iothalamate as a contrast medium (Telebrix, Byk Gulden, Constance).

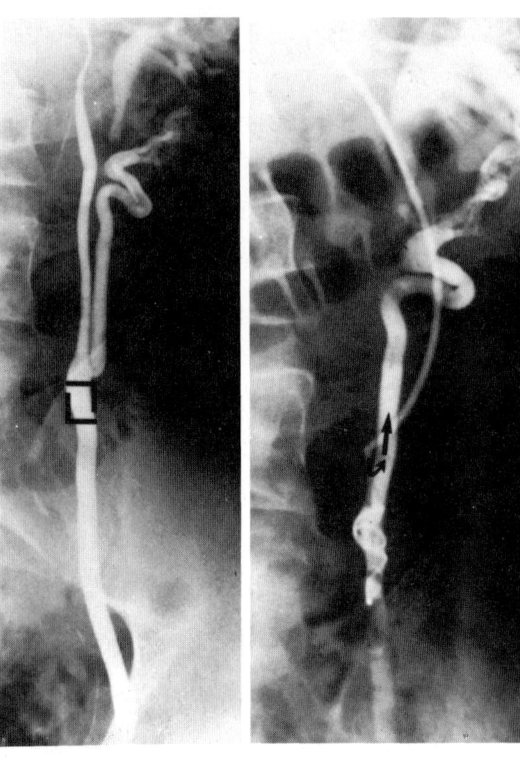

a

b

Fig. 1. a Retrograde phlebography of testicular vein (with central bifurcation). b Occlusion by spiral below the bifurcation. Thrombosis 12 min following occlusion not yet complete. Contrast medium is carried off via the duplicate central vein (arrows). The distal part is visualized only weakly

For the purpose of occlusion, the diagnostic Seldinger catheter (Oedmann-Ledin catheter 7 F) has to be replaced by the special set of Gianturco embolization instruments. A guide wire previously introduced into the testicular vein serves as a "guard rail" for the catheter, whose internal diameter permits the passage of the spiral. In order to achieve the required position of the catheter tip, it is sometimes necessary to use guide wires of different stability. Moreover, it can be useful to change the position of the patient and have him carry out various breathing maneuvers. At the moment of embolization, the catheter tip must be introduced into the vein at least one spiral length (extended spiral = 6 cm). The spiral is introduced into the catheter by means of a special mandrin and a special guide wire. As soon as the spiral is pushed out of the catheter tip, it rolls up and takes its predetermined form.

For the first two embolizations we used two spirals; however, a 20 min observation showed that 1 spiral is sufficient for complete occlusion. If possible, the spiral is placed in the region of the iliosacral joint since there is less movement of the trunk in this segment than in the upper lumbar part and, consequently, dislocation of the spiral may be avoided.

Patients

The method described was performed on 24 patients suffering from varicocele requiring therapy. The existence of varicocele was verified by clinical examination, plate thermography, and a phlebogram; a spermiogram was made in every case.

Short-term Results

After embolization, the catheter was left in the central part of the testicular vein for more than 20 min. The site of embolization was examined by means of test injections at intervals of about 10 min (Fig. 2). There was a progressive thrombosis, which was complete after about 20 min. In two patients, a control phlebogram was made 2 days after embolization (Fig. 3); the testicular vein was occluded centrally. (Long-term results, see L. Weissbach et al., this symposium).

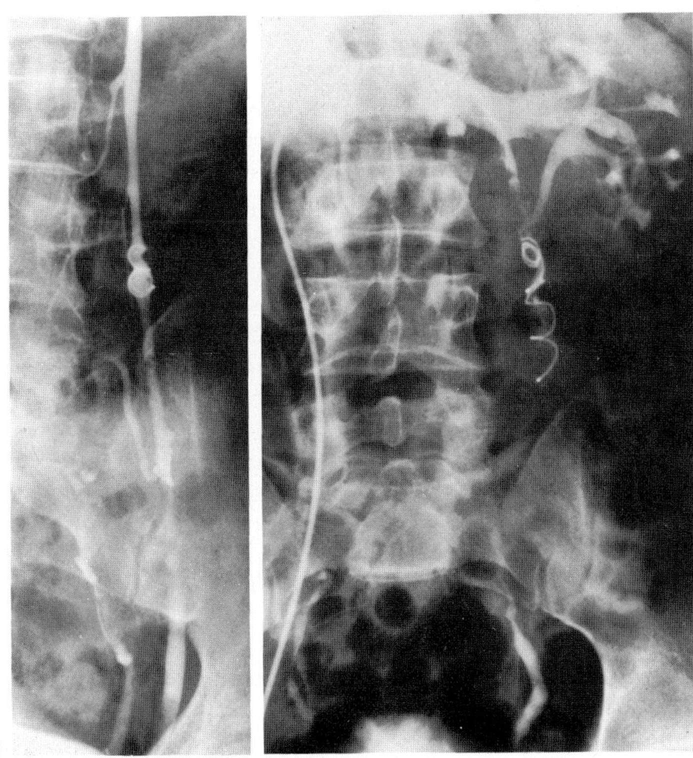

Fig. 2. Retrograde phlebography 10 min following embolization employing a spiral, which is seen closely above the left iliosacral joint. Due to the width of the spiral, the testicular vein bulges slightly. Partial flow of contrast medium into the distal venal parts

Fig. 3. Retrograde phlebography 2 days following embolization employing two spirals. Complete thrombosis of the central testicular vein has been achieved

Acute Complications

After application of the spiral, three patients had a gripping sensation in the left flank for 1–2 days. In one patient, these complaints lasted more than a week, then disappeared gradually. In another patient, a second spiral was introduced without regard for leaving a safe distance between the tip of the embolization catheter and the renal vein (length of the extended spiral was 6 cm), so that the last turn of the spiral penetrated into the lumen of the renal vein. Extraction by surgical intervention was necessary. At the time of the in situ examination, the testicular vein, where the first spiral remained, was completely thrombosed. After an observation period of 10 days, the patient was discharged without complaints; there were no further acute complications.

Critique of the Method

In our experience, there are two conditions on which an embolization therapy is not feasible:

1. The testicular vein or a collateral circulation cannot be clearly probed; in such cases, the embolization catheter cannot be placed safely. This is the case, for instance, if the descending testicular vein is very tortuous.
2. The diameter of the vein to be embolized is superior to that of the rolled-up spiral. In such cases, the spiral may be dislocated and pushed into the renal vein and the pulmonary circulation.

Moreover, the method cannot be applied if the varicocele is on the right side; in fact, the right testicular vein can be probed and represented angiographically only in exceptional cases. It is probably seldom possible to introduce the embolization catheter deeply enough and still keep a safe distance from the inferior vena cava.

Furthermore, the method is contraindicated if the pathologic filling of the pampiniform plexus is not due to valvular insufficiency of the testicular vein or its collateral veins, but to anastomoses between the external iliac vein and the testicular vein, with inverted flow of blood.

Discussion

Except for the said limitations, the embolization of idiopathic varicocele is an alternative to traditional therapy, especially when surgical intervention was unsuccessful.

Since phlebography and subsequent treatment are possible without accompanying medication, there is no general anesthesia, no surgical intervention, and no necessity for the patient to stay in hospital for 5–10 days. The method requires but little equipment; all that is needed is an angiographic catheter instrumentarium, a special set of instruments for embolization, and an image-intensifying television system. A roentgenoscope is preferable to an angiographic unit because it allows the patient to be in a semi-upright position. This is useful for the angiographic representation of varicocele; the insufficient venous system and inverted flow of blood can be seen more clearly. The time required for diagnostic phlebography and subsequent occlusion therapy is 45–60 min, including preparations. This is comparable to the time required for surgical interventions. The rate of persistency of varicocele results from the possible existence of collateral vessels and variants of vascular course and discharge. These findings emphasize the importance of phlebography, which permits an elective embolization therapy.

It is true that, for the new embolization method, a 5-day observation period in hospital is still advisable; however, increasing experience will probably permit a reduction of this time.

The drawbacks of our method are the application of a foreign body and the rate of complications resulting from diagnostic phlebography. However, the V2A alloy that the embolization spiral is made of does not differ from other implantable foreign bodies, which do not provoke any reactions. The appearance of short- or long-term side effects of practical importance may be the scattering in the position of the spiral (cf. L. Weissbach et al., this symposium). Occlusion of the testicular vein by means of the Gianturco spiral should be performed whenever the sclerosing method of obliteration is impossible or unsuccessful. With the latter procedure, no foreign body is left implanted.

Summary

The transcutaneous embolization therapy of idiopathic varicocele, which is based in the Seldinger catheterization technique, is an alternative to the well-known surgical methods, in which the rate of persistency or relapse is said to be between 0% and 25%. For our new variant of transcutaneous catheter embolization we use the Gianturco spiral. The spiral embolization can be done subsequent to a diagnostic transfemoral phlebography of the left testicular vein, which permits us to determine the indication or contraindication of the method. Our method has been applied to 24 patients who suffered from a varicocele which required medical therapy.

References

1. Iaccarino V (1977) Trattamento conservatio del Varicoceles: Flebographia selettiva e Scleroterapia delle vene gonadiche. Riv Radiol 17:107
2. Lima SS, Castro MP, Costa OF (1979) A new method for the treatment of varicocele. Andrologia 10/2:103
3. Riedl P (1979) Varikozelen-Verödung. Muench Med Wochenschr 121/5:157
4. Riedl P (1979) Selektive Phlebographie und Katheterthrombosierung der Vena testicularis bei primärer Varikozele. Wien Klin Wochenschr [Suppl] 91:99
5. Thelen M, Weissbach L, Franken Th (1979) Die Behandlung der idiopathischen Varikozele durch transfemorale Spiralokklusion der Vena testicularis sinistra. ROEFO 131:24
6. Thelen M, Weissbach L, Franken Th (1980) The treatment of idiopathic varicocele by transfemoral spiral occlusion of the vena testicularis sinistra. In: Percutaneous biopsy and therapeutic vascular occlusion. Thieme, Suttgart New York, pp
7. Zeitler E, Jecht E, Herzinger R, Richter E-I, Seyferth W, Grosse-Vorholt R (1979) Technik und Ergebnisse der Spermatika-Phlebographie bei 136 Männern mit primärer Sterilität. ROEFO 131:179
8. Zeitler E, Jecht E, Richter E-I, Seyferth W (1980) Selective sclerotherapy of the internal spermatic vein in patients with varicoceles. In: Percutaneous biopsy and therapeutic vascular occlusion. Thieme, Stuttgart New York, pp 190–193

Treatment of Varicoceles by Embolization with Detachable Balloons
Abstract

K. H. Barth, S. L. Kaufman, S. Kadir, and R. I. White, Jr.

Detachable silicone balloons were used in 11 patients to embolize the testicular vein draining a varicocele. Ten patients had a unilateral left varicocele and one patient had right and left varicoceles. In the latter patient both varicoceles were occluded in the same session. Typically the testicular vein draining the right varicocele entered the right renal vein. Following initial testicular venography, the optimal place for balloon detachment was selected. One occlusive balloon was required in eight embolizations and two balloons in four embolizations. The four patients requiring two balloons for embolization either had duplication or branching of the testicular vein. All but one varicocele remained effectively treated through the 10 months of follow-up. The one recurrence was the left varicocele in the patient with the bilateral varicoceles. Follow-up angiography revealed occlusion of the proximal portion of the left testicular vein even after the balloon had spontaneously deflated. The varicocele was apparently sustained by pelvic collaterals.

The technique of detachable balloon embolization of varicoceles briefly consists of transfemoral catheterization of the testicular vein with a coaxial catheter system. The outer catheter is nontapered 9 F (3 mm ϕ) o.d. and is advanced into the proximal testicular vein. A venogram is then performed to outline the venous anatomy. This is followed by injection of the balloon catheter and balloon positioning in the desired area. The balloon is then inflated to a maximum of 0.4 ml with a maximum diameter of 9 mm. Proper balloon fit is checked before detachment.

This method appears to represent a highly selective, well-controlled, and effective way of treating scrotal varicoceles as an alternative to surgical ligation. It can be performed as an outpatient procedure. The testicles are excluded from direct X-ray exposure during fluoroscopy and venography, and measured testicular doses did not exceed 50 mrem.

Nonsurgical Cure of Varicocele by Transcatheter Embolization of the Internal Spermatic Vein with Bucrylate

M. KUNNEN

Introduction

In 1975–1976 we described a method for selective retrograde venography of the internal spermatic vein [3, 4] which is now widely used all over the world [1, 2, 6, 7, 9]. After having examined more than 350 patients suspected of primary varicocele by means of transfemoral, selective retrograde venography of the internal spermatic vein, a new method was developed for the nonsurgical cure of this disease, i.e., embolization with the tissue adhesive isobutyl 2-cyanoacrylate (IBC_2, Bucrylate from Ethicon).

To date, we have treated 40 patients, of whom 3 had bilateral varicoceles. The technique is safe, relatively simple, and certainly successful. The diagnostic venography and subsequent embolization are performed on an outpatient basis. The method is neither painful nor stressing for the patient, who leaves the department cured of his disease.

Method

The embolization is performed exclusively using coaxial catheters, a set of which is manufactured by Surgimed S. A., Denmark (4465 TPB 070 and 15100A012) according to the author's instructions.

The outer catheter (7.2 F) is typically cobra-shaped and is at first used for diagnostic venography. This examination is performed from the right groin under local anesthesia and without any other (pre)medication.

The venography must be carried out carefully in order to demonstrate not only the pathologic, retrograde filling of the internal spermatic vein, but also all accompanying, connecting, or collateral veins. Based on the venographic findings, the ideal site of embolization is exactly localized. The site must be situated inferior to the lowest anastomosis between the spermatic vein and the renal or perirenal venous plexus (Figs. 1 and 2). The procedure is only performed if the spermatic vein shows no parallel veins at the site of embolization. Ramifications occurring superior or inferior to the level of embolization are then of no importance.

Immediately after the selective venography has been performed, a thin inner catheter (3.3 F), fitted with a suitable guide wire (Cook TSF 21125), is pushed through the diagnostic cobra-catheter into the internal spermatic vein. During this procedure the tip of the guide wire reaches slightly out of the thin catheter. All catheters are continuously moistened with glucose 5% through a T-adaptor.

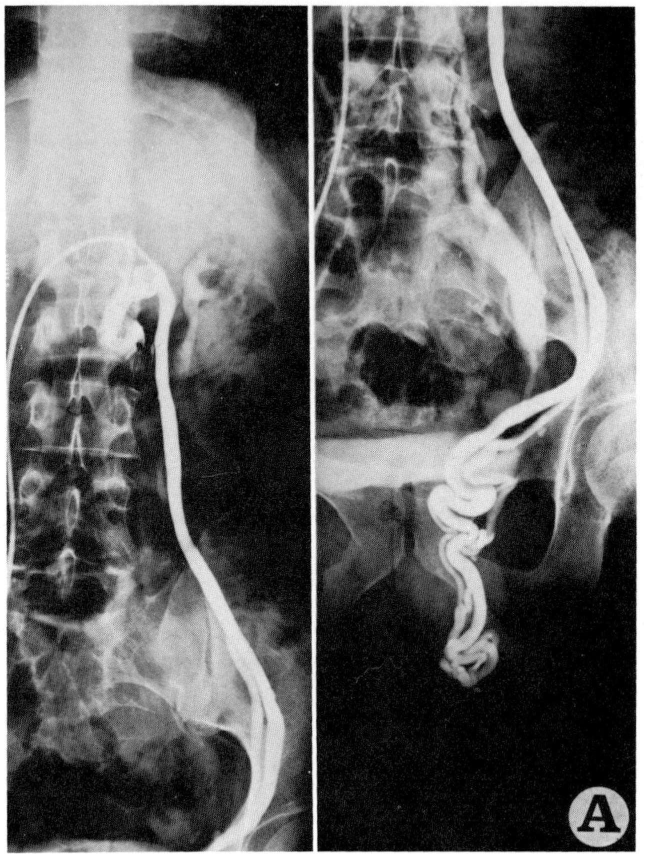

Fig. 1A–C. Case 1. Embolization with IBC₂ of a bifurcated left internal spermatic vein. **A** Diagnostic venogram visualizing a large left-sided varicocele. **B** Control venogram performed 10 min after embolization. The thrombosis is not yet complete. **C** The control venogram 30 min after embolization and during forceful Valsalva maneuver demonstrates that total occlusion is achieved

Under fluoroscopic control, the tip of the inner catheter is brought to the exact site elected for embolization. The catheter moves more easily when the patient performs a Valsalva maneuver.

After the guide wire is removed, a few milliliters of Isopaque 60% are injected by hand in order to control the exact localization of the catheter. The patient is brought into a nearly horizontal position (2°–5°) C in order to stop the blood circulation in the spermatic vein. Accidental thrombosis of the renal vein becomes impossible and injection in the testicular veins is equally excluded.

A first tuberculin syringe is filled with 1 ml glucose 10%. In a second syringe the following substances are aspirated in sequence: first, 0.1 ml Isopaque 60%, then be-

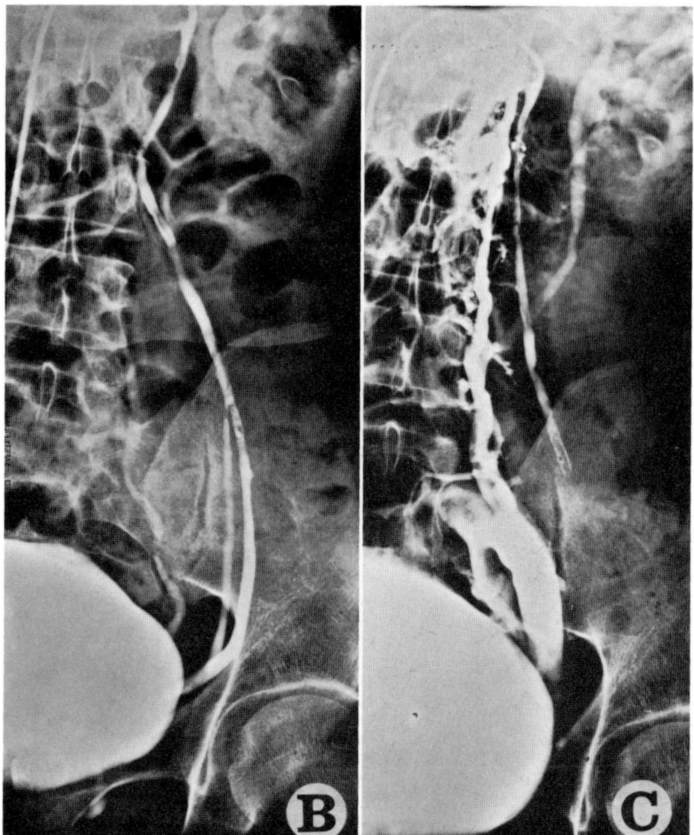

Fig. 1 B–C

tween 0.3 and 0.6 ml IBC$_2$, and finally another 0.1 ml Isopaque 60%. The contents of the second syringe are injected into the embolization catheter and pushed into the spermatic vein by means of the contents of the first syringe. Indeed, 0.7 ml glucose 10% is injected to push the embolus totally into the spermatic vein. As the coaxial embolization catheter is immediately pulled back (for 2 or 3 cm), the remaining 0.3 ml glucose 10% is injected in order to completely clean this catheter of bucrylate. The inner catheter is then withdrawn. The outer cobra-catheter is pulled back into the caval vein and rinsed with glucose 5%. If any resistance is noticed while doing so, the adherence of a IBC$_2$ residue is suspected, and the outer catheter is also withdrawn. This, however, should not normally occur. As soon as the tissue adhesive comes in contact with blood, it polymerizes to form a thrombus.

About 10 min later, a control venography is performed using the cobra-catheter. First, the renal vein is injected without a Valsalva maneuver to check its integrity. The renal vein is then injected during a Valsalva maneuver, and finally the thrombosed spermatic vein is selectively visualized.

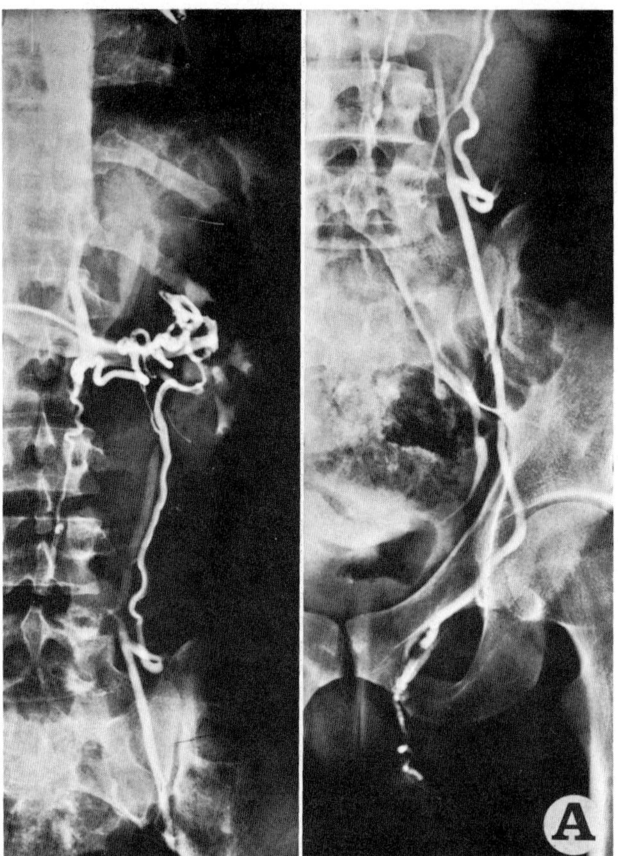

Fig. 2A–C. Case 2. Diagnostic venography in a patient with varicocele and competent valves
in the cranial part of the left internal spermatic vein, but presenting reflux through a bypassing
collateral into the caudal part of the vein. **A** Left side renal venogram: a competent valve is
shown at the outlet of the internal spermatic vein. A tortuous, insufficient collateral stands out
clearly. It bypasses between a caudal segmentary renal vein and the insufficient caudal segment of the internal spermatic vein. **B** Enlargement demonstrating more clearly the anastomosis. **C** Reflux can be forced during selective catheterization of the internal spermatic vein,
the cranial valve becoming incompetent; the second valve remains competent (*arrow*)

Patients

Up to now, the procedure has been performed on 40 patients with a left-sided
varicocele. Three of these patients had previously been operated on without success.
Three patients presenting bilateral varicoceles were treated at both sides.

The varicoceles were detected by clinical examination, thermography, and/or
Doppler flow measurement (reference Comhaire et al., this book). Spermiograms
were performed in all cases.

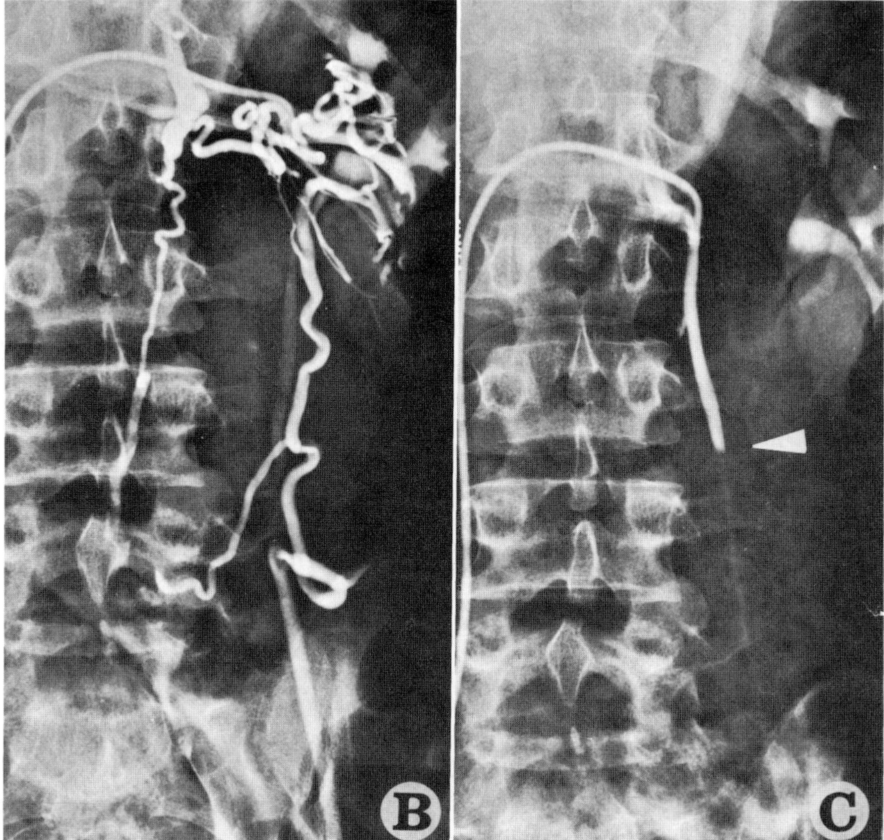

Fig. 2 B–C

Results

In 33 cases a total occlusion was found on the control venography performed 10 min after embolization; five cases took 30 min to occlude completely (Fig. 1), whereas in two cases a second dose of 0.3 ml IBC_2 had to be given during the same session in order to obtain complete obliteration.

At the start of our studies we used glucose 20% to push the embolus, and this probably caused a too-slow polymerization of the IBC_2, resulting in an incomplete occlusion. Since we use 1 ml glucose 10% and a sufficient quantity of IBC_2, complete thrombosis is obtained immediately.

In all cases a control examination showed disappearance of reflux on clinical palpation and on either thermography or Doppler flow measurement. Control hormonal measurements and spermiograms presented encouraging improvement; half of the men treated for more than 6 months succeeded in impregnating their wives.

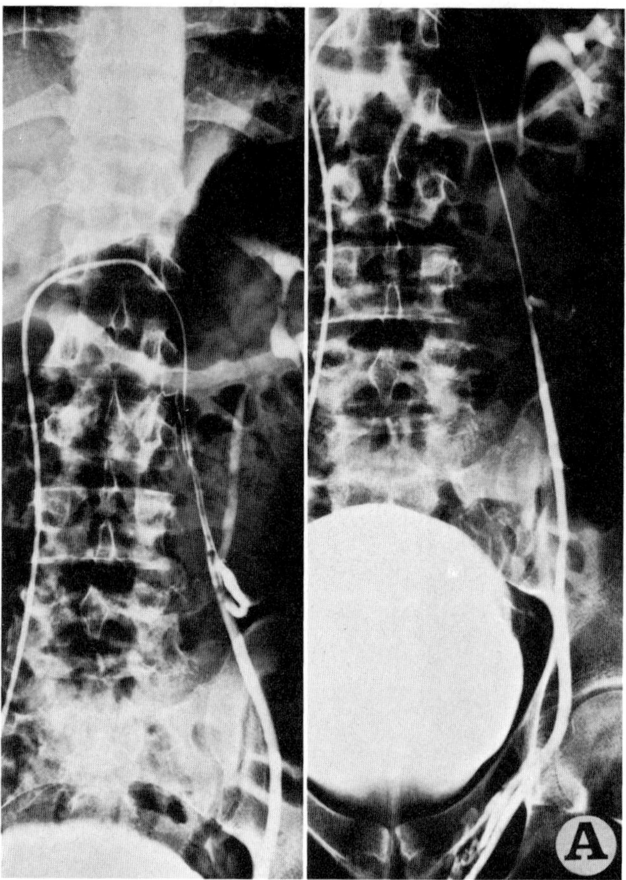

Fig. 3 A–C. Case 2. Embolization with IBC$_2$ in the same patient as **Fig. 2. A** The small inner catheter (3.3 F) has passed several competent valves, the tip is situated caudal to the bypassing anastomosis with the segmentary renal vein. **B** The embolus is injected in the spermatic vein. The caudal limit of the embolus is clearly outlined by means of Isopaque 60% (*arrow*). **C** Control left side renal venogram demonstrating a total occlusion of the internal spermatic vein caudal to the anastomosis (*arrow*). (The opacified ureter slightly disturbs the venogram)

One patient was operated on for right-sided inguinal hernia 3 months after embolization. During this operation, an ascending venography of the left spermatic vein was performed which disclosed a total occlusion at the exact site depicted on the control descending venography performed immediately after embolization.

Complications

The patients have no complaints at all during, as well as after, the embolization procedure. Examination and treatment are performed on an outpatient basis. One

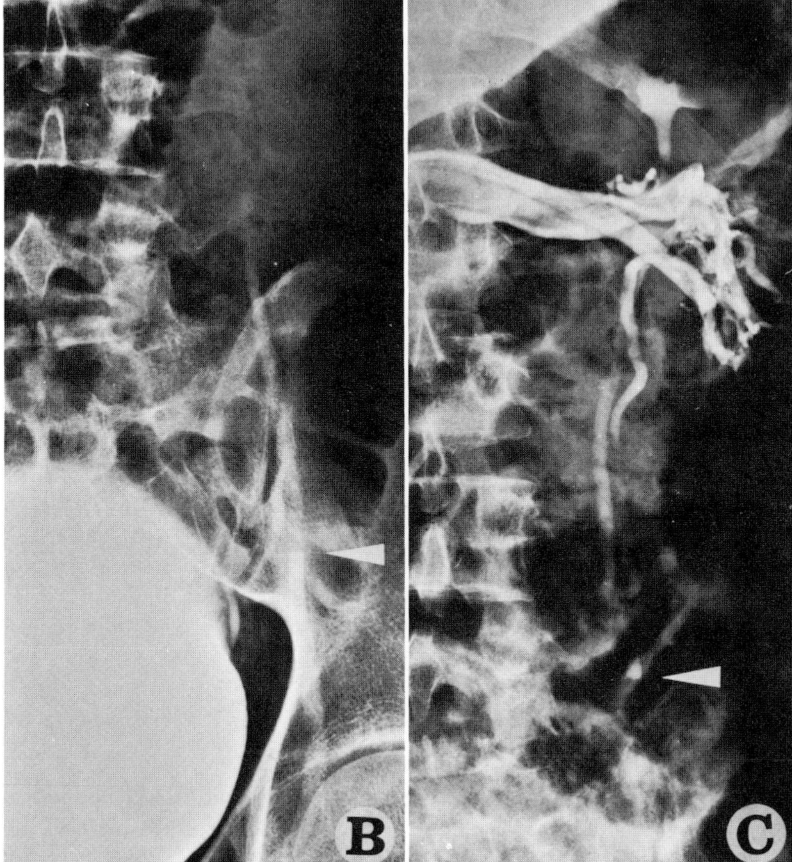

Fig. 3 B–C

single incident occurred in the third case treated. In this man the coaxial catheter was not pulled back immediately and after less than 3 min it was found to be trapped in the embolus. The patient was operated on and recovered uneventfully.

Discussion

Treatment of primary varicocele by selective embolization of the internal spermatic vein is safe, successful, and relatively simple. From results published on IBC_2 application for arterial occlusion [5] and for obliteration of the gastric coronary vein and esophageal varices [8], it is known that the obliteration is definitive. Only a mild histiocytic foreign body, giant cell reaction is found in the vessel 2–196 days after embolization. No ischemic or inflammatory complications were ever observed after application of isobutyl 2-cyanoacrylate. Such reactions frequently occurred after methyl 2-cyanoacrylate treatment; therefore this product is to be discarded. Zanetti and Sherman [11] and Freeny et al. [5] have demonstrated that no more than 15% of the Bucrylate cast is actually in contact with the vessel endothelium. The tissue adhesive forms a sponge-like matrix which entraps red blood cells in its interstices. After 2 months the interstices become densely fibrotic and contain histiocytes and foreign body giant cells. This reaction is, however, clearly confined to the lumen of the vessel and does not involve the vessel wall or contiguous tissues.

Care should be taken to use glucose 5% solution as a rinsing and moistening fluid since a sodium chloride solution would induce precocious polymerization of the IBC_2. Furthermore, one should only use disposable plastic catheters and syringes.

In our hands the method has no disadvantages. However, it requires an experienced angiographic facility and careful application. It appears that even large veins can be embolized without problems; this is not possible with the Gianturco spiral [10]. The latter technique cannot be used in cases presenting reflux through collateral veins and competent valves in the cranial part of the spermatic vein. With our method it was possible to pass through several competent valves and to successfully embolize the insufficient caudal part of the spermatic vein (Figs. 2 and 3).

The obliteration using bucrylate embolus can be localized more selectively than with sclerotherapy [7, 9]. Using IBC_2, one is absolutely certain that no drug will enter the blood circulation, and that no contact with the testis will occur. Pain, thrombophlebitis, or extravasations indeed never occurred in our patients.

Conclusion

Bucrylate treatment performed without general anesthesia and on an outpatient basis presents outstanding advantages over conventional methods for varicocele treatment.

References

1. Bigot JM, Chatel A, Dectot H, Hélénon Ch (1978) Phlébographie spermatique rétrograde. Ann Radiol (Paris) 21:515–523
2. Chatel A, Bigot JM, Hélénon Ch, Dectot H, Rotman J, Salat-Baroux J (1978) Intérêt de la phlébographie spermatique dans le diagnostic des stérilités d'origine circulatoire (varicocèle). Ann Radiol (Paris) 21:565–570
3. Comhaire F, Kunnen M (1976) Selective retrograde venography of the internal spermatic vein: a conclusive approach to the diagnosis of varicocele. Andrologia 8:11–24
4. Comhaire F, Monteyne R, Kunnen M (1976) The value of scrotal thermography as compared with selective retrograde venography of the internal spermatic vein for the diagnosis of "subclinical" varicocele. Fertil Steril 27:694–698
5. Freeny PC, Mennemeyer R, Kidd CR, Bush WH (1979) Long-term radiographic-pathologic follow-up of patients treated with visceral transcatheter occlusion using isobutyl 2-cyanacrylate (Bucrylate). Radiology 132:51–60
6. Janson R, Weissbach L (1978) Zur Phlebographie der Vena testicularis bei Varikozelenpersistenz bzw. -rezidiv. ROEFO 129:485–490
7. Lima SS, Castro MP, Costa OP (1978) A new method for the treatment of varicocele. Andrologia 10:103–106

8. Lunderquist A, Börjesson B, Owman T, Bengmark S (1978) Isobutyl 2-cyanoacrylate (Bucrylate) in obliteration of gastric coronary vein and esophageal varices. Am J Roentgenol 130:1–6
9. Riedl P (1979) Selektive Phlebographie und Katheterthrombosierung der Vena testicularis bei primärer Varikocele. Wien Klin Wochenschr [Suppl] 91:99
10. Thelen M, Weissbach L, Franken Th (1979) Die Behandlung der idiopathischen Varikozele durch transfemorale Spiralokklusion der Vena testicularis sinistra. ROEFO 131:24–29
11. Zanetti PH, Sherman FE (1972) Experimental evaluation of a tissue adhesive as an agent for the treatment of aneurysms and arteriovenous anomalies. J Neurosurg 36:72–79

Modified Technique for Embolization of the Internal Spermatic Vein

Ch. L. Zollikofer, A. Formanek, W. Castaneda-Zuniga, and K. Amplatz

Insufficiency and absence of the valvular apparatus in the spermatic veins is one of the major causes of male infertility. One out of every six couples in the United States is infertile [5]. In 25% of male patients with an abnormal spermiogram no varicocele is palpable, but an incompetent internal spermatic vein can be demonstrated on spermatic venography [4]. Therefore, bilateral spermatic venography is indicated as a diagnostic test, since no varicocele may be palpable and anatomic variations are common [6, 7, 8].

The conventional transfemoral technique has two drawbacks. First, the right internal spermatic vein especially can be catheterized only with difficulties and, second, it may be impossible to advance the catheter into the periphery for safe embolization. Therefore, we developed the transjugular approach, which allows selective catheterization of both spermatic veins with demonstration of the anatomy and subsequent embolization which can be carried out in the same sitting.

Materials and Methods

Thirteen male patients from 25 to 37 years of age with a history of infertility and a pathologic spermiogram underwent bilateral spermatic venography after thorough physical examination. Venography was performed regardless of a clinically detectable varicocele, provided the patient had an abnormal spermiogram. The percutaneous transjugular approach was used. In ten patients embolization was attempted after demonstrating a varicocele or incompetent spermatic vein.

Technique of Venography

The right internal jugular vein is punctured 5–6 cm above the level of the right clavicle (Fig. 1). Once the vein is punctured, a gently curved french size 7 or 8 catheter (Fig. 2) with a braided wire mesh is introduced into the inferior vena cava. In most cases (85%) the right spermatic vein enters the inferior vena cava along the right anterolateral wall [2], at the level of L-1 to L-2 vertebrae. This catheter can be readily advanced deep into the right spermatic vein unless competent valves are present (Fig. 3).

If the right spermatic vein arises from the renal vein (in approximately 7%–10% of the cases) [2, 7], the same catheter can be easily introduced deep into the right renal vein and pulled back along its inferior wall to enter the right spermatic vein (Fig. 3).

The same technique and catheter is used for the left spermatic vein. By slowly withdrawing the catheter tip along the inferior aspect of the left renal vein, the left spermatic vein is entered (Fig. 3). If this catheter fails, a modified "head-hunter" is

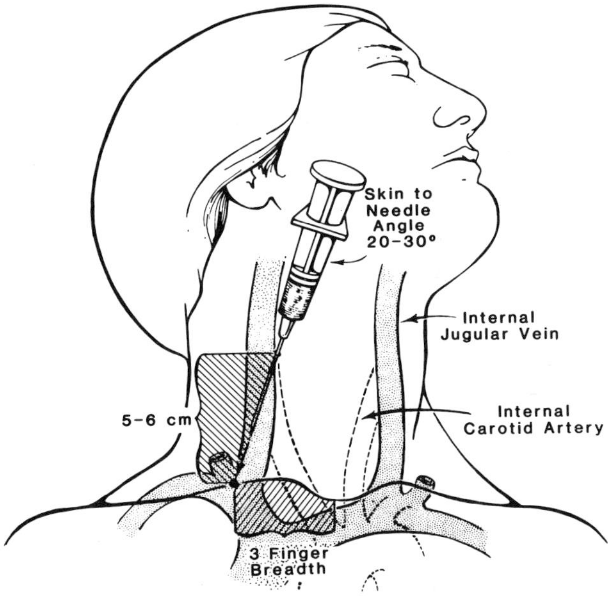

Fig. 1. The patient's head turned 45° to the left facilitates the location of the puncture site. The anatomic relation and the direction of the needle is demonstrated. The angle between the needle and the skin of the neck should be 20°–30°

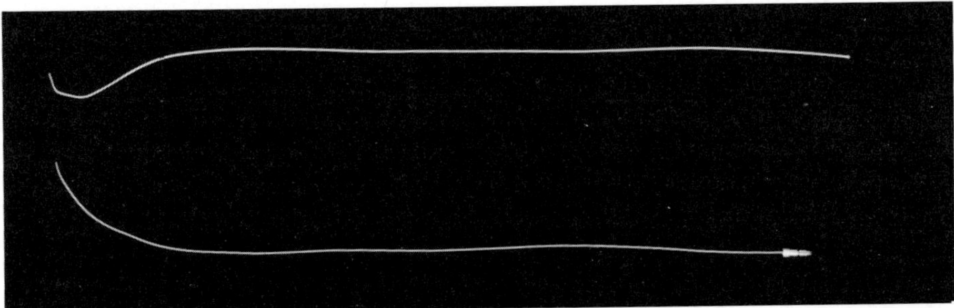

Fig. 2. The distal portions of the catheters used for selective catheterization of the spermatic veins via transjugular approach are shown. The catheter in the upper part is used for both the right and left spermatic vein; the catheter in the lower part is used for the left spermatic vein only if the slightly J-shaped catheter fails to enter the left spermatic vein selectively

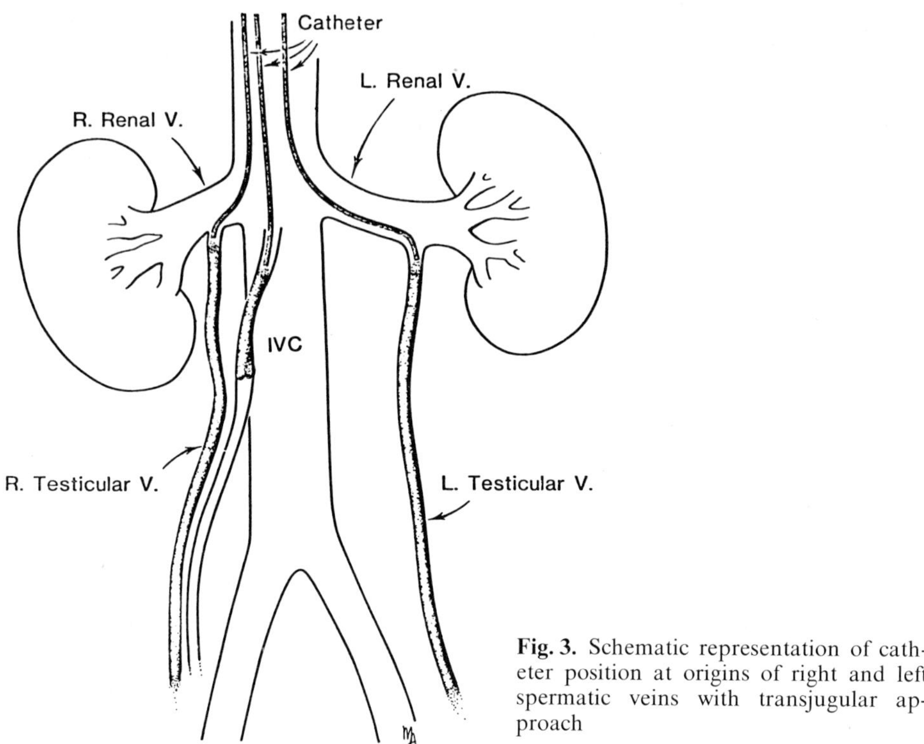

Fig. 3. Schematic representation of catheter position at origins of right and left spermatic veins with transjugular approach

used for left-sided spermatic venography (Fig. 2). Once the spermatic vein is entered the catheter can be advanced over a guide wire. Spermatic venography is carried out both with and without a Valsalva maneuver to demonstrate the incompetent spermatic vein or varicocele.

Embolization Technique

Occlusion of the spermatic vein is carried out according to the angiographic findings. At least one additional obstructing device is placed as close as possible to the level of the renal vein (Fig. 4). This prevents the potential hazard of dislodgement of long thrombi and pulmonary embolism. For embolization we used stainless steel coils with or without Dacron tails[1] and compressed Ivalon plugs[2]. Both occluding devices are easily introduced through a thin walled straight 0.110 OD catheter[3]. The diameter of the coils has to be significantly larger than the diameter of the spermatic vein to prevent embolization of the coil. The coils can be advanced deeply into the spermatic vein beyond the level of the catheter tip by a technique recently reported by us [1].

---

1 Gianturco coils, Cook Incorporated
2 Scientific Apparatus Shop, University of Minnesota
3 Formacath, Becton-Dickinson, Rutherford N.J.

Ivalon is compressed around a special introducing wire. A stainless steel spring wire is slipped over this introducing wire as a means to strip off and deliver the Ivalon plug (Fig. 5). This system is rapidly advanced through the catheter under fluoroscopic control. The plug is extended beyond the catheter tip and positioned at its desired location. Upon contact with blood the plug expands to the original 8–9 mm in diameter and causes permanent occlusion (Figs. 6–8). The plug can now be stripped off with the spring wire and the introducing wire together with the spring wire is pulled out (Figs. 6–8). The technique has been described previously in detail [9].

Until organization of the Ivalon plug occurs, only pressure of the expanding plug against the wall of the spermatic vein holds the plug in place. This represents a potential hazard for embolization. Therefore, a large coil or steel umbrella is placed downstream to the expanded plug (Fig. 9). Because animal experiments demonstrated that steel coils may get dislodged, we now routinely use stainless steel umbrellas also after embolization with coils (Figs. 10, 11).

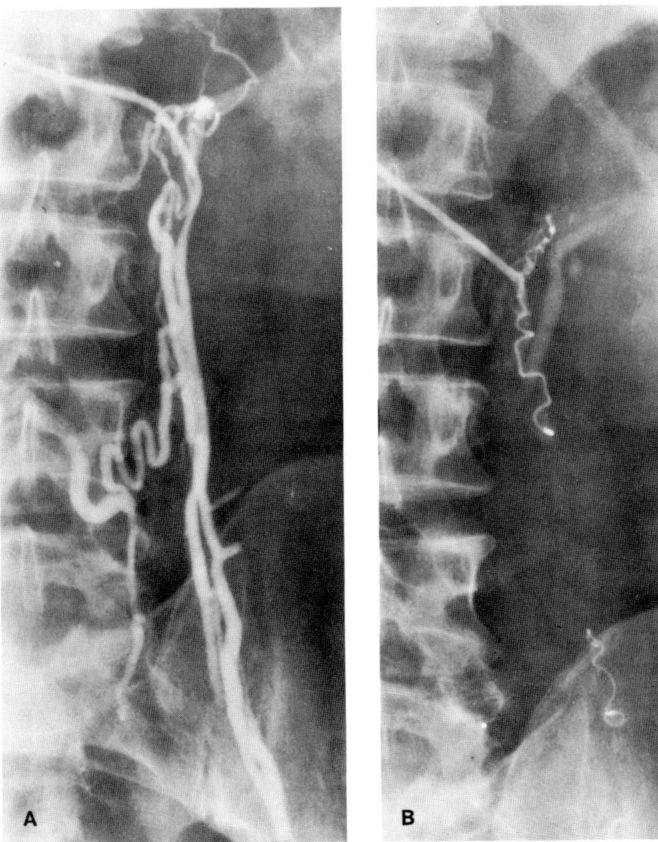

Fig. 4A and B. Left varicocele with collaterals of the proximal spermatic vein (**A**) requiring placement of occluding devices proximally and distally to collateral vein (**B**). Also note proximal coil close to renal vein preventing a large thrombus

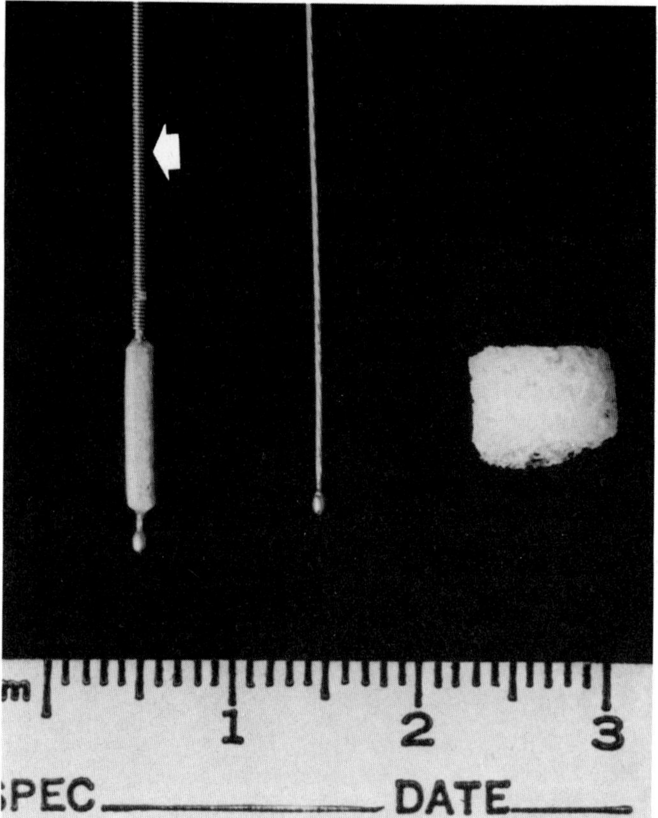

Fig. 5. *Right,* Expanded Ivalon plug 8 mm in diameter. *Middle,* Special introducing wire. *Left,* Ivalon plug after compression around introducing wire. Note spring wire behind Ivalon plug (*arrow*)

Fig. 6 A and B. Right spermatic venogram (transfemoral approach) showing right-sided varicocele

Fig. 7. A Ivalon plug (nonradiopaque) compressed around tip of introducing wire (*arrow*) is positioned beyond catheter tip (*arrowhead*) (transjugular approach; same patient as in **Fig. 6**). **B** After expansion of Ivalon plug the introducing wire and spring wire are pulled back

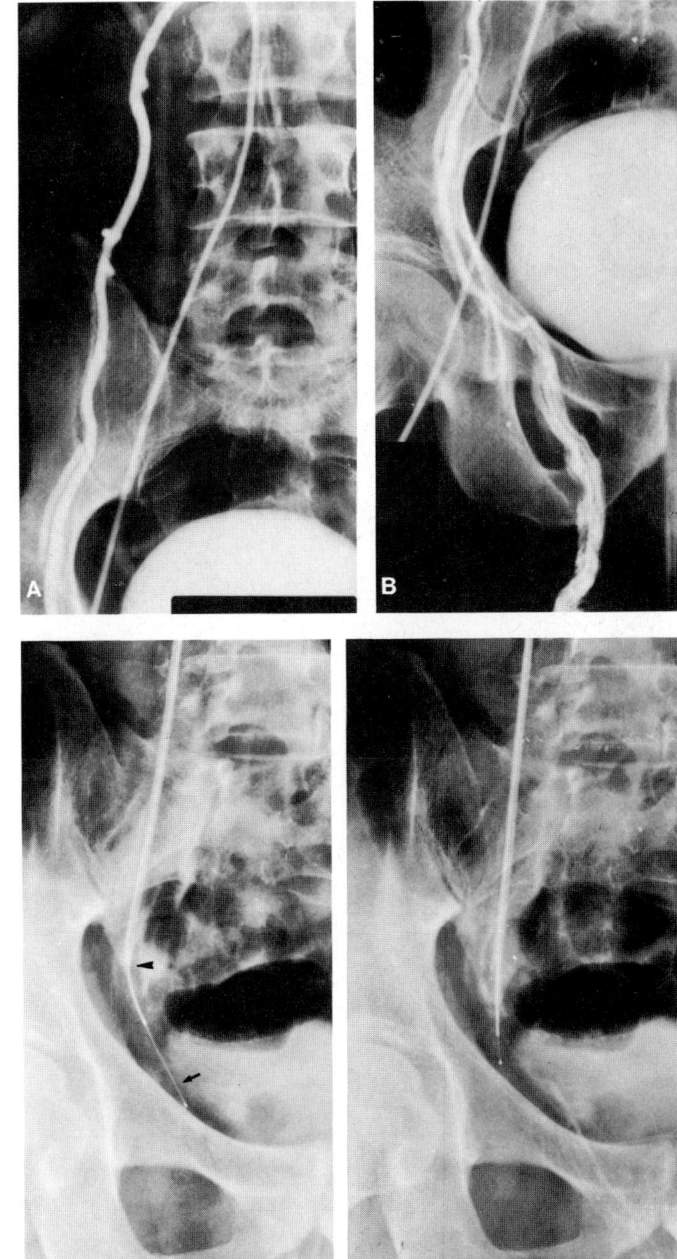

Fig. 6 A, B

Fig. 7 A, B

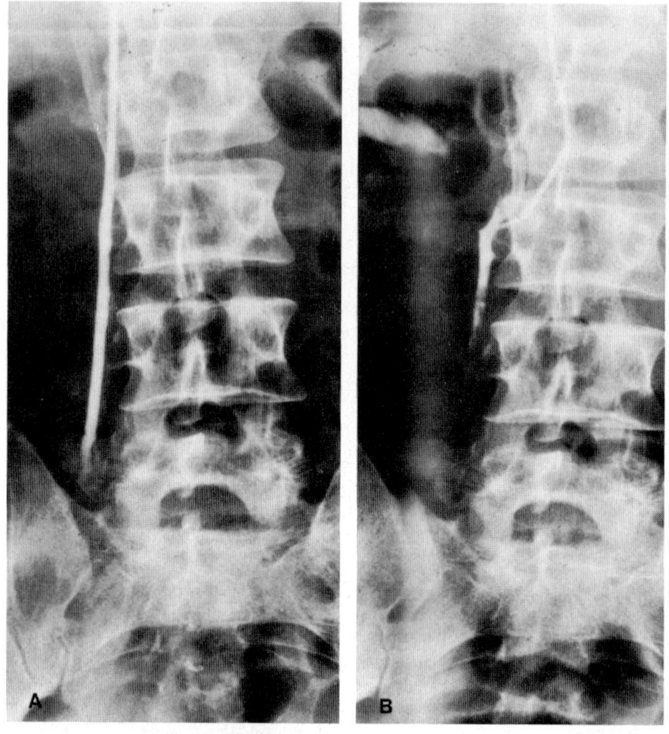

Fig. 8 A, B

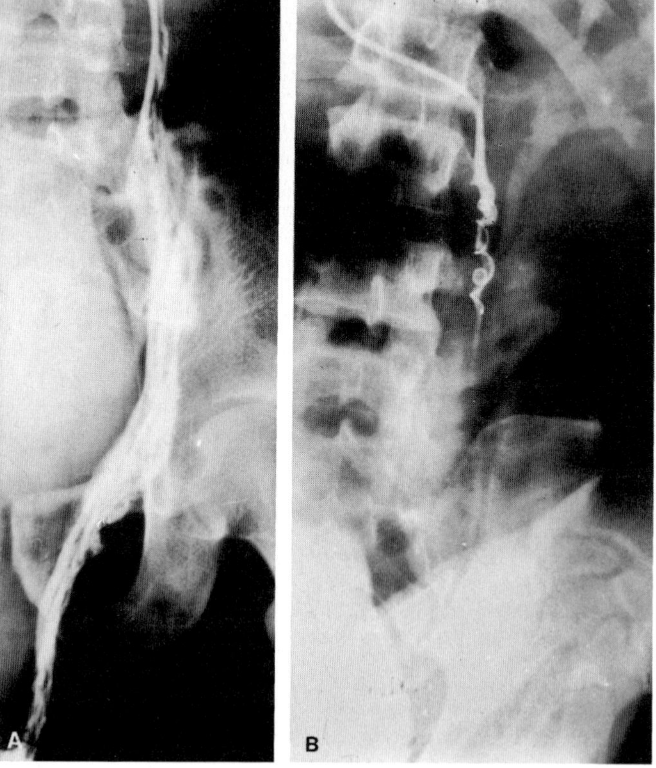

Fig. 9 A, B

Fig. 10. Embolization of left varicocele with coils. A stainless steel umbrella (*arrow*) was placed downstream to the coils to prevent dislodgement. There is some extravasation of contrast due to catheter manipulation

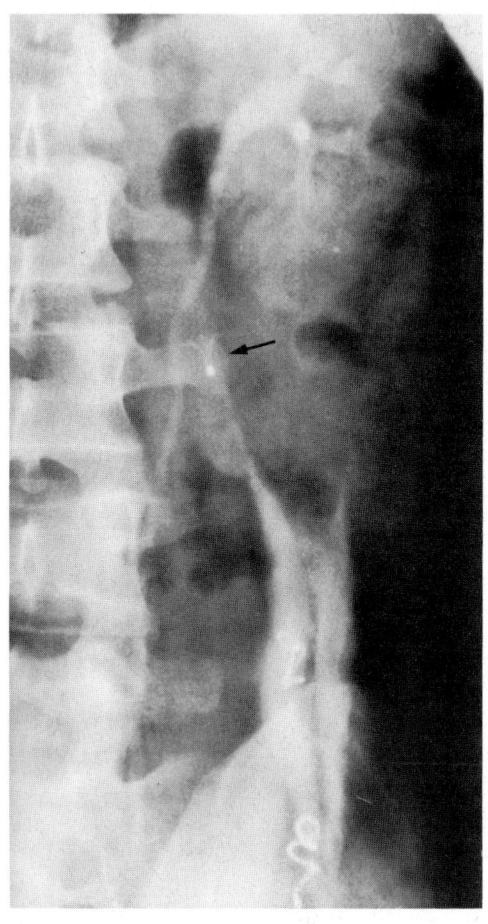

Fig. 8. A Control venogram after placement of two Ivalon plugs in the pelvic region. There is complete occlusion of the right spermatic vein at the pelvic rim (same patient as in **Figs. 6, 7**). **B** Control venogram after placement of a third Ivalon plug in the proximal right spermatic vein

Fig. 9. A Spermatic venogram showing left varicocele. **B** Complete occlusion after embolization with two Ivalon plugs. A coil was placed downstream to expanded plugs to prevent potential dislodgement of Ivalon plugs

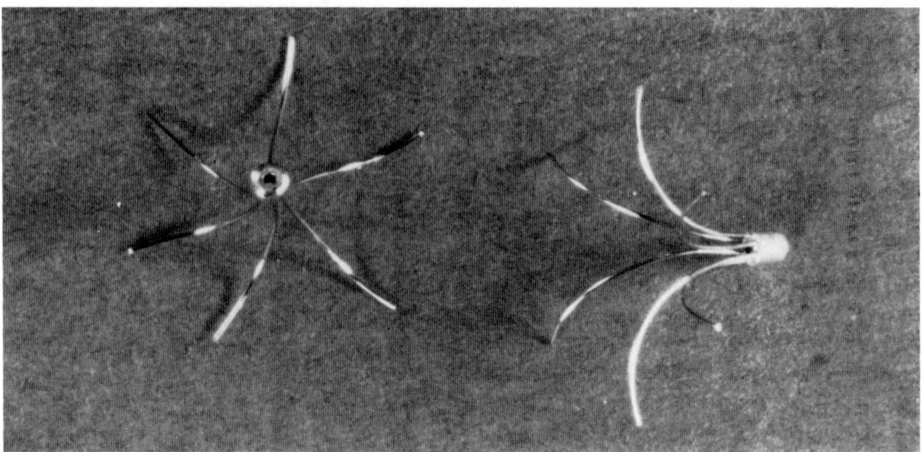

Fig. 11. Close up view of stainless steel umbrella that can be inserted through the selective catheter

Results and Discussion

Our experience with 13 patients may be summarized as follows (Table 1).

In all 13 patients there were no difficulties in catheterization of the left spermatic vein. In one of these patients the previously ligated spermatic vein was demonstrated. In two patients, anatomic variation with anomalous origin of the left spermatic vein from a small intrapelvic branch of the renal vein precluded safe embolization. In the remaining ten patients, embolization was carried out successfully with coils or Ivalon plugs.

In 11 patients, catheterization of the right spermatic vein was attempted with only one failure. In all ten patients successfully catheterized, right spermatic veins valvar incompetence with reflux was demonstrated. We therefore believe that valvar incompetence is probably always bilateral in spite of only a clinically left-sided varicocele. In eight cases the right spermatic vein was successfully embolized. In the remaining two patients, recatheterization of the spermatic vein following venography was not possible due to spasm or subintimal injection of contrast medium.

Total occlusion of the spermatic vein with Ivalon plugs or coils without Dacrontail required 5–10 min and was documented by venography (Figs. 4b, 8b, 9b).

Our preliminary results with the new transjugular approach indicate that embolization of both spermatic veins can be achieved with consistency. The internal jugular vein approach allowed successful catheterization of the internal spermatic veins in 23 of 24 attempts and successful embolization was accomplished in 18 of 20 cases (Table 1). It was surprising to find in almost all cases an associated right-sided spermatic vein incompetence. This finding raises the question of a bilateral congenital valvar insufficiency. This was also confirmed by Chatel, who found incompetence of the right spermatic vein in 80% of patients with left-sided incompetence [3]. There were no serious complications except for breakage of a small catheter segment which embolized to a pulmonary artery branch. However, this event could oc-

Table 1. Results of selective catheterization of the spermatic vein and their nonsurgical occlusion in 13 patients with transjugular approach

Number of attempts for selective catheterization	number of successes	number of interruptions with occlusive devices		Patients not having non-surgical interruption of the spermatic vein
		Successes	Failures	
Left sper-matic vein	13	13	10	0	One patient had surgical ligation of the left vein
					Two patients had anomalous origin of the vein precluding safe nonsurgical occlusion
Right sper-matic vein	11	10	8	2	In two patients after the initial venogram the veins could not be recatheterized because of spasm or extravasation of contrast medium
Total	24	23	18	2	

cur with any catheterization procedure. Venous spasm or perforation of the spermatic vein may occur but have no consequences.

The number of our patients treated with nonsurgical occlusion is limited as yet. However, follow-up spermatograms 4–6 months postocclusion showed significant improvement in sperm count and motility in three out of four patients.

Conclusions

The catheterization of the spermatic veins via transjugular approach is relatively simple. Especially for the selective catheterization of the right spermatic vein, this new method is easier than the conventional transfemoral method and rarely fails. The catheter can be advanced deeply into the spermatic veins, allowing a safe, nonsurgical occlusion on both sides. The procedure can be carried out on a ambulatory basis, which reduces costs.

References

1. Castaneda-Zuniga W, Zollikofer C, Barreto A, Formanek A, Amplatz K (to be published) A new device for the safe delivery of stainless steel coils. Radiology
2. Chatel A, Bigot JM, Dectot H, Helenon Ch (1978) Anatomie radiologique des veines spermatiques. Chirurgie 115:443–450
3. Chatel A, Bigot JM, Helenon Ch, Dectot H, Rotman J, Salat-Baroux J (1978) Interêt de la phlebographie spermatique dans le diagnostic des sterilites d'origine circulatoire (varicocele) Ann Radiol (Paris) 21:565–570

4. Comhaire F (1978) Extra testicular factors in male infertility. Acta Clin Belg 33:181–190
5. Howards SS, Lipshultz LI (1978) Symposium on male infertility. Forward. Urol Clin North Am 5:433–436
6. Janson R, Weilsbach L (1978) Zur Phlebographie der Vena testicularis bei Varikozelen-persistenz bzw. -rezidiv. ROEFO 129:485–490
7. Sabatier JC, Bruneton JN, Drouillard J, Tavernier J, Ducos M, Fleury B, Latapie JL (1977) Phlebographie spermatique: Techniques. Indications. Ann Radiol (Paris) 20:539–544
8. Zeitler E, Jecht E, Herzinger R, Richter EI, Seyferth W, Grosse-Vorholt R (1979) Technik und Ergebnisse der Spermatica-Phlebographie bei 136 Männern mit primärer Sterilität. ROEFO 131:179–184
9. Zollikofer C, Castaneda-Zuniga W, Galiani C, Formanek A, Amplatz K (to be published) Compressed ivalon: A new technique for deliveries.

D. Complications and Risks

Complications of Surgery for Varicoceles

L. V. WAGENKNECHT

In our experience, high ligation of the spermatic vein for varicocele is an operation with an extremely low incidence of complications and almost without adverse reactions. We have performed high ligation of the spermatic vein in 650 patients with idiopathic varicocele. There was a serious complication in only one patient, who suffered from postoperative hemorrhage and had to be reoperated upon. Subcutaneous bleeding occurred in 2%–3% of the patients and was easily treated by one or two stitches under local anesthesia. In two patients a hernia developed due to insufficiency of the sutures, requiring surgical intervention.

Late *sequelae* are hydroceles, which were found in approximately 2% of our patients 2–24 months after surgery but required no treatment. Celoids were treated by plastic surgery. A persistent varicocele following high ligation of the spermatic vein was evident in 5 of the 633 patients[1]. Postoperative persistence of varicoceles is due to overlooked branches of the spermatic vein and collaterals to the presacral, paravertebral, perirenal, and pampiniform plexus or to the iliac and femoral vein. In conclusion, high ligation is a safe and simple surgical technique.

---

1 see page 133

Complications and Risks of Percutaneous Sclerotherapy and Gianturco coil Embolization

E.-I. RICHTER and E. ZEITLER

Like each angiographic or phlebographic procedure, phlebography of the internal spermatic vein also involves a certain number of contrast media reactions. The contrast media quantity applied varies between 40 and 80 ml; sometimes 150 ml are necessary for double-sided demonstration.

Only 1 of the 419 patients we treated suffered an immediate contrast media reaction. This patient had a known tetania. The questions, however, as to what extent hyperventilation was responsible for the acute symptomatology remained unanswered. The acute symptoms disappeared after oxygen respiration and intravenous injection of calcium. The patient was supervised for 24 h and further reactions were not observed.

Slight contrast media reactions, e.g., nausea, sensation of heat, sudation, urticaria, spot-shaped erythema, manifested in 4% of the examined patients. These symptoms quickly disappeared after oxygen respiration, application of corticosteroids (Urbason, Solu Decortin), and injection of antihistamines (Fenistil, Tavegil) and sometimes calcium, additionally.

Intraarterial application of local anesthetic must be avoided. We had one such a case: a patient submitted to control phlebography after sclerotherapy suffered a disorientation for a short time.

Small hematomas in the pelvis seldom occur, and only in cases of unintended arterial puncture. Phlebothromboses in the leg or pelvis were not observed in our patients who underwent control phlebography after sclerotherapy, and were neither observed nor reported from other teams. All follow-up controls manifested an entirely patent pelvic vascular system.

Paravascular and subintimal contrast media application is the most frequent concomitant symptom besides the contrast media reaction during phlebography and sclerotherapy of the internal spermatic vein. More often this was observed when using sharp-edged catheters with tips bent beyond a right angle than those with less-angled tips. Sometimes subintimal location of the catheter could be avoided with industrial-made catheters.

A subintimal or paravascular contrast media application mainly occurs at the ostium of the left internal spermatic vein to the renal vein, peripherally in the spermatic vein with a selectively placed catheter, or in the caudal caval vein behind the ostium of the right internal spermatic vein.

A paravascular contrast media application can happen in one of the following ways:

a) With a narrow lumen of the internal spermatic vein.
b) With a too-high injection pressure during phlebography or application of sclerosing agent.
c) If, during application of contrast media or sclerosing agent the patient exerts a too-forceful Valsalva maneuver, and the selectively placed catheter tip then cannot avoid the counterpressure.

Normally, the paravascular contrast media was absorbed within 1 h; on discharge of the patient 2 h later only a small remaining amount of contrast media distributed indistinctly around the original puncture site might be seen, but this entirely disappears within 24 h. Sometimes patients noted a slight dragging pain in the flank; we saw this in two cases. Only one did we have a perforation of the internal left spermatic vein during sclerotherapy.

As the sclerosing agent acts both intravascularly and extravascularly, one should give up sclerotherapy when perforating the internal spermatic vein since a fibrosis in the retroperitoneal space, possibly near the ureter, can theoretically occur. Whether the intravascular sclerosing effect exerts an influence on the retroperitoneal space, too, is unknown but improbable.

Sclerotherapy of the right internal spermatic vein must be given up particularly in cases of paravascular application of contrast media because the internal spermatic vein and ureter cross and a fibrosis must be avoided around the ureter in the retroperitoneal space.

Despite these objections and the incidents which theoretically may occur, we must emphasize that such occurrences have not been observed so far. If, however, perforation of the internal spermatic vein occurs, sclerotherapy should immediately be discontinued. In certain circumstances, however, perforation alone might be a sufficient reason that an occluding thrombosis develops.

A side effect of varying intensity that nearly all patients noted during sclerotherapy was a dragging pain in the course of the internal spermatic vein. Sometimes it radiated into the left side. The reason might be the efflux of sclerosing agent into other supply veins in the spermatic vein. This pain, however, abates within a few minutes and when the patient is discharged 2 h later, it has disappeared. Nevertheless, we recommend all patients to apply a suspensory and a cold compress in case pain recurs in the course of the spermatic vein in the abdomen or testicles. Two patients who developed a local thrombophlebitis in the testicles within 24 h had to use these measures and the symptoms disappeared in the following 2 days.

Follow-up controls after sclerotherapy revealed a varix in the testicles of five patients. In the meantime, one of these patients reported that infertility has been corrected.

Occlusion of the internal spermatic vein is a special problem when applying the sclerosing agent. In patients with a very wide internal spermatic vein, the balloon catheter can successfully be placed in the vein and efflux of sclerosing agent avoided.

In a very narrow internal spermatic vein with a selectively placed catheter, the catheter itself already has an occluding effect. Nevertheless, a minor efflux of sclerosing agent might occur in these cases and in others in which occlusion with the balloon catheter is abandoned.

Follow-up control of the contrast media application and irritations of taste that patients note show that such an efflux of sclerosing agent occurs. This is the reason why patients' posture should be variable during application of sclerosing agent. If the occlusion is nearly complete, the patient remains in a horizontal position during application. If, however, occlusion of the veins is incomplete or not secured, the patient is placed in an oblique position under the fluoroscope with his head elevated at 30°–45°.

The risk of such an efflux of sclerosing agent – less than 1–2 ml – is still uncertain. Side effects other than taste irritations were not observed. Moreover, follow-up controls showed that at no time was a thrombosis produced in the renal vein after sclerotherapy. The question must be left open as to whether the sclerosing agent that flows in a small and considerably diluted quantity through the renal vein, the caudal caval vein, and the heart into the pulmonary circulation might be harmful.

In our clinic we have no experience in occlusion treatments with the Gianturco coil or detachable balloons and therefore possible complications can be discussed only theoretically.

The Gianturco coil is a metal device placed into the vein against the blood flow. We know from intraarterial application where embolization takes place with the blood flow that, very seldom, due to flow effects or mechanical manipulations, a spiral might enter the aorta or the renal artery on the opposite side. This, however, is significant in the arterial system. The consequences of a displacement of the metal spiral from the internal spermatic vein over the renal vein into the caudal caval vein are unclear, as are the consequences of a displacement and transport over the right heart into the pulmonary circulation. Introduction of a spiral is very simple and produces a local thrombosis in the spermatic vein. To what extent, however, the intravascular metal spiral causes an additional fibrosis in the retroperitoneal space after thrombosis has not yet been investigated.

The risks involved in the location of a detachable balloon for occluding the internal spermatic vein are equally unclear. Theoretically, one can assume that a location of a balloon in the vein against the blood flow is much more doubtful than the location of a spiral.

On the other hand, a balloon which has left the vein with the blood flow can easily be perforated anywhere with a spiral during a subsequent catheterization, its diameter thus being reduced. Moreover, the contrast-filled balloon spontaneously contracts by itself. Therefore, we think that the general risk is lower with a detachable balloon than with a metal spiral. On the other hand, it is possible that reactions produced by balloon occlusion in the retroperitoneal space are inferior to that of a metal spiral. This, however, is a purely theoretical assumption, since own experiences with both procedures are lacking.

Risks and complications of sclerotherapy arise from contrast material application which, incidentally, might occur during each phlebographic procedure and from a possible allergic reaction. Patients are therefore supervised for 2 h after treatment to keep any complications under control. Finally, such complications that occur during an occlusive treatment with embolization material, must be avoided. The risk involved in sclerotherapy is confined to the site of application of the sclerosing agent. Simultaneous occlusion of parallel and multiple side branches of the internal spermatic vein – which might be the basis for recidivation – is another considerable advantage of sclerotherapy and cannot be produced by local occlusion, be it ligature, balloon catheter treatment, or occlusion with spiral.

A fatal or severe risk has not yet occurred. Further development of this treatment procedure, however, involves complications and one should be prepared right from the beginning to control them.

References

1. Iaccarino V (1980) A non surgical treatment of varicocele: transcatheter sclerotherapy of gonadal veins. Ann Radiol 23:369–370
2. Janson R, Weissbach L (1978) Zur Phlebographie der V. testicularis bei Varikozelenpersistenz bzw. -rezidiv. Fortschr Röntgenstr 129:485
3. Riedl P (1979) Selektive Phlebographie und Katheter-Thrombosierung der Vena testicularis bei primärer Varicocele. Wien Med Wochenschr 91 [Suppl 99]
4. Thelen M (1980) Embolization in Varicoceles. Symposium "Perkutane Biopsie und therapeutische Vasookklusion" 1979. Anacker H (Hrsg) Thieme, Stuttgart New York

VI. Results

Long-Term Results after Surgical Treatment of an Idiopathic Varicocele

J. Haselberger, L. Knebel, and G. Ludwig

Improved results in the spermiogram, as well as a raised rate of conception after surgical treatment of an idiopathic varicocele, are reported by numerous authors [1, 3, 8a, 10, 23, 27, 33, 36, 38, 41]. Results concerning the extent and the time of the improvement after operation largely agree, but are in some cases varying to divergent. Several authors consider that an improvement of the spermiogram occurs above all within the 1st year after the operation and that afterwards the spermiogram deteriorates again. This suggests that it would be advisable to operate on a varicocele only when conception is intended to take place within the next year.

On the other hand, other study groups such as that of Boeminghaus et al. [2], Hornstein [15], Maus et al. [27], Weissbach et al. [41], Hienz et al. [14a] advocate as we do that varicoceles should also be eliminated in adolescents and children as a prophylactic andrological measure against possible future fertility disorders. This procedure appears appropriate since it is precisely the long-term results after surgical treatment of an idiopathic varicocele that are of special importance.

Results

Between 1971 and 1979, 164 idiopathic varicoceles were operated on with high partial resection of the internal spermatic vein branches according to Bernardi at the University Department of Urology in Mannheim. Of the idiopathic varicoceles, 97% had appeared on the left side. This is to be explained on the basis of anatomical and pathophysiological factors which have been described in detail in the literature [7, 9, 14, 14a, 15, 19, 24, 40].

Follow-up examinations could be made in 99 of the 164 patients operated on. Of these 99 patients, 72 had had the operation at least 1–5 years previously. These 72 patients were considered in the discussion of the long-term results. The remaining 27 patients, who had been operated on within the past year, were also given a follow-up examination. However, by definition they could not be accounted to the long-term results.

The age distribution of the patients at the time of the operation is as follows: children and adolescents (7–16 years old), 32 patients (19.5%); adults (18–46 years old), 132 patients (80.5%).

As mentioned above, we had established the indication for varicocele operation in children and adolescents as prophylaxis against possible fertility disorder. We established the indication in adults when there was a pathological spermiogram and in a normal spermiogram when there was a sterile marriage with a desire for children. We were somewhat more cautious in establishing the indication for surgery because of local symptoms based on a varicocele, since experience shows that freedom from symptoms can be achieved only in a certain percentage.

Possible causes of pain in varicocele patients, in the form of a pulling pain in the affected half on the scrotum radiating into the groin, are either the varicocele itself, traction on the venous plexus, or a venous congestion in the testis. Pain is also due to an inguinal hernia, which is by no means uncommonly found in addition. The latter was often only developed as incipient hernia or "weak groin". One cannot expect any improvement by a surgical elimination of the varicocele when a genital femoral nerve neuralgia is involved. We observed this three times with simultaneous idiopathic varicocele.

Our follow-up examinations comprised inspection and palpatory examination of the body, exclusion of urinary tract infections, and preparation of a spermiogram. In the patients with markedly pathological spermiograms, a control spermiogram was set up in all cases. As usual, sexual abstinence for five days was required.

The literature data on the improvement in the spermiogram after varicocele operation is listed in Table 1 and contrasted with our own long-term results in the 72 patients who were followed up. The criteria of the spermiogram improvement in this listing concern both spermatozoan density *and* motility.

Table 1. Spermiogram improvement after varicocele operation (spermatozoan density and motility)

Author	No. of varicocele operations	Spermiogram improvement in %
Afflerbach et al. [1]	10	90
Boeminghaus et al. [2]	95	84
Weissbach [40]	35	83
Dubin and Amelar [8]	111	81
Kaufmann et al. [16]	80	80
Dubin and Hotchkiss [9]	88	75
Völter et al. [39]	23	73
Dubin and Amelar [8 a]	504	71
Scott and Young [35]	166	70
Kolle et al. [21]	34	70
Charney [5]	36	64
Pontennier et al. [30]	21	62
Charney and Baum [6]	104	61
Tulloch [37]	30	60
Brown et al. [4]	185	60
Schellen and Canton [32]	25	60
Gasser [13]	29	59
Brown [3]	295	58
Cohen et al. [7]	19	33
Klein [17]	62	31
Own patient material (long-term results)	72	80

Afflerbach et al. [1] reported an improvement of semen quality in 92% of their patients following varicocele operation. However, the number of patients followed up by these investigators [1] was only ten. In contrast, Klein [17] found an improvement of semen quality in only 31% of his patients operated upon.

Most authors report values between 60% and 70%. We ourselves found a long-term improvement of 80% in our 72 cases, as did Boeminghaus et al. [2], Weissbach [40], Dubin and Amelar [8], and Kaufmann et al. [16].

If one breaks down the improvement of the spermiogram separately according to the rise in the spermatozoan density and improvement of motility as is done in Table 2, only a limited correlation between the improvement of the spermatozoan density and improvement of motility is shown. The spermatozoan density, reported with values between 16% by MacLeod in 1969 [26] and 78% by Scott in 1961 [34], fluctuates very much more strongly than the motility after the varicocele operation, although ranges of variation between 50% and 80% were also found here.

In our own long-term results we found a rise of the spermatozoan density in 51% and a rise of the motility in 62% (Table 2).

Table 2. Spermiogram improvement after varicocele operation (comparison of spermatozoan density with motility)

Author	No. of varicocele operations	Rise of spermatozoan density (%)	Rise of motility (%)
Scott [34]	93	78	81
Scott and Young [35]	142	69	65
Fritjofsson and Ahren [11]	35	62.5	50
MacLeod [25]	77	61	63
Pauwels et al. [29]	20	55	50
MacLeod [26]	108	16	74
Own patient material (long-term results)	72	51	62

Table 3. Varicocele persistence (according to various authors)

Author	No. of varicocele operations	Persistence (%)
Palomo [28]	40	0
Robb [31]	40	2.5
Fritjofsson et al. [12]	44	11.3
Fritjofsson und Ahren [11]	37	5.4
Klosterhalfen and Schirren [18]	55	0
Gasser [13]	51	7.8
Knöner and Dathe [20]		13.0
Lindholmer et al. [22]	20	25.0
Klosterhalfen et al. [19]	519	0.96
Own patient material	72	6.9

Although conclusive evidence for the biological significance of the individual spermiogram parameters is still lacking, most authors consider that motility is more important for fertility than is spermatozoan density.

We found an unchanged or even impaired spermiogram after varicocele surgery in 14 of 72 cases, i.e., roughly 20%. We were able to identify as possible causes a varicocele persistence in one case, an epididymitis which had run its course in another case, a subsequently performed bilateral herniotomy in a third case, and a testicular parenchymal lesion verified by biopsy with substantial tubulus fibrosis in a fourth case. The cause remained unclear in the other ten cases. However, we do not have any testicular biopsies from these cases and it is entirely possible that the damage to the germinal epithelium due to the varicocele was already so great that irreparable damage had occurred.

Varicocele persistences were found in five of the 99 patients who were followed up. However, only one of these had a pathological spermiogram. Four patients showed a normal spermiogram; the varicocele appeared to have thrombosed 3 months postoperatively in all cases. However, a recurrence (even if less pronounced), or more precisely, a persistence, was observed in the further course.

Our 5 persistences in 72 cases correspond to a persistence rate of 6.9%. As can be seen from Table 3, persistence rates between 0% and 25% are reported in the literature.

Summary

The long-term results after surgical elimination of a varicocele according to Bernardi are very good; the overall spermiogram is improved in 80% of cases. There is a differentiated 51% rise of spermatozoan density and 62% rise of motility. These are better than the earlier results in which we were only able to observe an overall improvement of about 40% during the first year after the operation.

The results support the thesis that a varicocele should be operated on not only in the presence of a pathological spermiogram and desire for children, but also with regard to preventing a possible later lesion to the testicular parenchyma.

References

1. Afflerbach F, Gaca A, Macher E (1968) Die idiopathische Varikozele als Ursache von Fertilitätsstörungen und ihre Behandlung durch hohe Unterbindung von A. und V. spermatica. Dtsch Med Wochenschr 93:2427
2. Boeminghaus H, Kollias G, Haensch R (1973) Subfertilität und Varikozele. Z Urol 66:443–449
3. Brown JS (1976) Varicocelectomy in the subfertile male. Fertil Steril 27:1046
4. Brown JS, MacLeod J, Hotchkiss RS (1969) Results of varicocelectomy in subfertile men. Exhibit at the 25th Annual Meeting of the American Fertility Society, Miami
5. Charny CW (1962) Effects of varicocele on fertility. Fertil Steril 13:47
6. Charny CW, Baum S (1968) Varicocele and Infertility. JAMA 204:1166
7. Cohen MS, Plaine L, Brown JS (1975) The role of internal spermatic vein plasma catecholamine determinations in subfertile men with varicoceles. Fertil Steril 26:1243

8. Dubin L, Amelar RD (1970) Varicocele size and results of varicocelectomy in selected subfertile men with varicocele. Fertil Steril 21:606

8a. Dubin L, Amelar RD (1975) Varicocelectomy as therapy in male infertility. Fertil Steril 26:217

9. Dubin L, Hotchkiss RS (1969) Testis biopsy in subfertile men with varicocele. Fertil Steril 20:50

10. Etriby A, Girgis SM, Hefnawy H, Ibrahim AA (1967) Testicular changes in subfertile males with varicocele. Fertil Steril 18:666

11. Fritjofsson A, Ahren C (1967) Studies on varicocele and subfertility. Scand J Urol Nephrol 1:55

12. Fritjofsson A, Ahlberg NE, Bartley O, Chidekel N (1966) Treatment of varicocele by division of the spermatic vein. Acta Chir Scand 132:200

13. Gasser G (1971) Varicocele. Wien Klin Wochenschr 26:484

14. Haensch R, Hornstein O (1968) Varikozele und Fertilitätsstörungen. Dermatologia 136:335

14a. Hienz HA, Voggenthaler J, Weissbach L (1980) Histological findings in testes with varicocele during childhood and their therapeutic consequences. Eur J Pediatr 133:139

15. Hornstein O (1964) Zur Klinik und Histopathologie des männlichen primären Hypogonadismus. Hodenparenchymschäden durch Varikozele. Arch Klin Exp Dermatol 218:347

16. Kaufmann J, Klosterhalfen H, Schirren C (1974) Operative Therapie der Verschlußaspermie und der idiopathischen Varikozele. Urol Int (Basel) 29:184

17. Klein PM (1971) Ergebnisse der operativen Therapie bei Infertilität des Mannes. Verh Dtsch Ges Urol 34:258

18. Klosterhalfen H, Schirren C (1968) Die operative Behandlung der Varikozele. Chir Praxis 12:425

19. Klosterhalfen H, Schirren C, Wagenknecht LV (1979) Pathogenese und Therapie der Varikozele. Urologe [A] 18:187

20. Knöner H, Dathe G (1971) Verbesserung der Ergebnisse der Varikozelenoperation durch präoperative Serienphlebographien. Verh Dtsch Ges Urol 25:335

21. Kolle P, Vogel PG, Fuchs R (1971) Indikation und Ergebnisse der hohen Ligatur der spermatischen Gefäße nach Palomo. Verh Dtsch Ges Urol 23:250

22. Lindholmer G, Thulin L, Eliasson R (1975) Semen characteristics before and after ligation of the left internal spermatic veins in men with varicocele. Scand J Urol Nephrol 9:177

23. Ludwig G, Jentzsch R, Peters HJ (1974) Fertilität bei idiopathischer Varikozele. Fortschr Med 31:1235–1239

24. Ludwig G, Jentzsch R, Peters HJ, Fiene R (1975) Die Klappen der Vena spermatica. Act Urol 6:89

25. MacLeod J (1965) Seminal cytology in the presence of varicocele. Fertil Steril 16:735

26. MacLeod J (1969) Further observations on the role of varicocele in human male fertility. Fertil Steril 20:545

27. Maus J, Schach H, Scheidt J (1974) Andrologische Untersuchungen bei subfertilen Männern vor und nach Varikozelenoperation. Hautarzt 25:394

28. Palomo A (1949) Radical cure of varicocele by a new technique. J Urol 61:604

29. Pauwels R, Festen C, Janknegt R, Moonen W (1970) Varicocelen subfertiliteit. Ned Tijdschr Genesskd 114:1565

30. Pontonnier F, Mansat A, Bennet P, Louvet L (1975) Varicocele et stérilité masculine (à propos de 71 observations). Rev Med Toulouse 11:323

31. Robb WAT (1955) Operative treatment of varicocele. Br Med J 2:355

32. Schellen TMCM, Canton M (1974) Varikozele und Subfertilität. Andrologia 6:330

33. Schirren C, Klosterhalfen H (1966) Die Spermatogenese bei Varikozele. Z Haut Geschlechtskr 40:372

34. Scott LS (1961) Varicocele: a treatable cause of subfertility. Br Med J 1:788

35. Scott LS, Young D (1962) Varicocele: A study of its effect on human spermatogenesis, and of the results produced by spermatic vein ligation. Fertil Steril 13:325

36. Steeno O, Knops J, Ceclerck L, Adimoelja A, van de Velde H (1976) Prevention of fertility disorders by detection and treatment of varicocele at school and college age. Andrologia 8:47
37. Tulloch WS (1955) Varicocele in subfertility results of treatment. Br Med J 2:356
38. Völter D (1971) Die idiopathische Varikozele aus andrologischer Sicht. Fortschr Med 90:683
39. Völter D, Knoth W, Lüders G (1971) Die Varikozelenoperation nach Giuliani. Dtsch Med Wochenschr 96:641
40. Weissbach L (1978) Die idiopathische Varikozele – Eine Übersicht. Extr Urol 1/3:255–268
41. Weissbach L, Hienz HA, Rodermund OE (1975) Spermatologische und histologische Befunde bei Patienten mit Varicocele. Urologe [A] 14:277

Spermatologic Results Preceding and Following Varicocele Surgery

G. Schieferstein and H. Kasseckert

The judgement of whether dysspermatogenesis is due to a varicocele cannot be performed objectively to date. One can detect various deviations from the norm of ejaculate parameters which have been found with more or less high frequency in often small groups of patients. Currently there is still a lack of extensive experience indicating the actual relevance of such deviations.

In studies of varying size, numerous authors have investigated the early and long-term effects of surgical treatment of varicoceles. Particularly in fluctuating populations, such follow-up studies encounter more difficulties the longer the period of investigation, i.e., the longer the period of time following intervention. The physiologic deviations in the spermiogram also constitute a factor of uncertainty which can be eliminated only to a certain degree.

We will present here the results of a follow-up investigation in which some of the above difficulties are particularly evident. The substantial fluctuation in the population of an industrial region with a high proportion of foreign residents and in the university town of Tübingen itself caused a greater reduction in the number of adequately monitored patients than we had expected. The significance of the present study was also reduced by other factors including the performance of the surgical interventions in different urologic departments, with different methods in some cases; postoperative examination of a portion of the patients by outside colleagues,

Table 1. Sperm *density* per milliliter before and after varicocele surgery

Before					$n = 84$	After				
0 – 1	1 – 10	11 – 20	21 – 40	> 40	$\cdot 10^6$/ml	0 – 1	1 – 10	11 – 20	21 – 40	> 40
9						5	3		1	
	33					2	16	6	5	4
		16					1	6	6	3
			13				1	2	3	7
				13				2	1	10
n 9	33	16	13	13	*n*	7	21	16	16	24
11%	39%	19%	15.5%	15.5%		8%	25%	19%	19%	29%

Unchanged $n = 40 = 47\%$
Deteriorated $n = 9 = 11\%$
Improved $n = 35 = 42\%$

Table 2. Sperm *motility* before and after varicocele surgery

Sperm density						Before				After			
						Total motility		Progr. motility		Total motility		Progr. motility	
0–1	1–10	11–20	21–40	> 40	$\cdot 10^6$/ml	< 70%	> 70%	< 40%	> 40%	< 70%	> 70%	< 40%	> 40%
9						9		9		9		8	1
	33					28	5	26	7	27	6	25	8
		⁄16				13	3	10	6	13	3	12	4
			13			12	1	10	3	11	2	8	5
				13		9	4	8	5	9	4	10	3
n 9	33	16	13	13	*n*	71	13	63	21	69	15	63	21
						85%	15%	75%	25%	82%	18%	75%	25%

Unchanged $n = 65 = 77\%$ $64 = 76\%$
Deteriorated $n = 9 = 11\%$ $10 = 12\%$
Improved $n = 10 = 12\%$ $10 = 12\%$

Table 3. Sperm *Morphology* Before and After Varicocele Surgery

Sperm density						before			after	
						normally shaped			spermatozoa	
0 – 1	1 – 10	11 – 20	21 – 40	> 40	· 10^6/ml	< 60%	> 60%		< 60%	> 60%
9						6	3		8	1
	33					23	10		17	16
		16				7	9		10	6
			13			3	10		2	11
				13			13		1	12
n 9	33	16	13	13	*n*	39	45	*n*	38	46
						46%	54%		45%	55%

Unchanged $n = 64 = 76\%$
Deteriorated $n = 10 = 12\%$
Improved $n = 10 = 12\%$

which means that all of the results did not originate from our department; and the availability of only one spermiogram from the period prior to or following surgery in a few cases. The follow-up investigations cover a postoperative period of 3 months to 5 years.

Due to the aforementioned reasons, we also cannot provide complete information on the actual success quotient, namely the subsequent pregnancies of the female partners following successful varicocele surgery.

The data of 84 patients operated upon in the years 1971–1979 turned out to be usable. Approximately 50% of the operations were performed in the last 3 years. The average age at the time of surgery was 31.5 ± 5.2 (21–45) years. Precise information on the length of time which the varicoceles had existed was not obtainable. In 82 patients (98%), a left-sided varicocele, and in two cases (2%), a bilateral

Table 4. Carnitine levels in seminal plasma before and after varicocele surgery

before									
sperm density						carnitine			
0–1	1–10	11–20	21–40	> 40	· 10^6/ml	< 4,5	4,5–10	> 10	mg/dl
1						1			
	9					8	1		
		3				2	1		
			7				5	2	
				3		1	1	1	
n 1	9	3	7	3	*n*	12	8	3	

varicocele was operated on. In six cases (7%), a hydrocele is known to have appeared after the varicocele operation and was later treated surgically. The indication for surgical treatment of a varicocele was determined separately from both the andrologic and urologic viewpoints. Patients were not eliminated due to additional factors which may have impaired spermiogenesis, such as existing hydroceles, earlier herniotomies or maldescension operations.

Results

Sperm Density (Table 1)

Prior to operation nearly 75% of the patients had a variously severe oligozoospermia, 11% cryptozoospermia or azoospermia. Only 15% had a sperm density exceeding 40 million per ml; most of these patients revealed motility disturbances.

Aside from slight deviations the postoperative sperm count per ml was unchanged in 40 patients (47%); i.e., these patients remained in the same relative class. Sperm density deteriorated in nine patients (11%) – with an approximate balance between those with variously marked oligozoospermia and those with normozoospermia. Sperm density increased in 35 cases (42%); broken down by individual classes, there was an increase in 44%–56% of the respective cases. If one draws a line at 20 million per ml, one can see that two-thirds of the patients were below the line prior to varicocele surgery and only about one-half of the patients after surgery.

Sperm Motility (Table 2)

We have broken motility down into total motility (percent of motile forms) with a normal value of more than 70% and progressive motility (forward motion) which normally should be exhibited by more than 40% of the spermatozoa.

Our results indicate that increased sperm density is linked with an improvement in motility. In 85% of the varicocele patients, however, motility was abnormal preoperatively, and progressive motility was disturbed in approximately three-quarters of the cases.

Table 4. Continued

after										
sperm density						carnitine			
0–1	1–10	11–20	21–40	>40	$\cdot 10^6$/ml	<4,5	4,5–10	>10	mg/dl
1						1			
	4	2	3			5	4		
	1	1	1			1	1	1	
		2	2	3			6	1	
		1		2			2	1	
n 1	5	6	6	5	n	7	13	3	

When considering the entire group of patients, surgical treatment of the varicoceles did not alter this situation. Though motility was normalized in 10 cases (12%), it deteriorated in nine or ten cases. The motility was unaffected by surgery in ca. 75% of the cases (Table 2).

Sperm Morphology (Table 3)

Similar to motility, the morphology of spermatozoa in varicocele patients reveals that sperm density correlates with the number of normally shaped spermatozoa. Whereas motility was disturbed in more than 75% of the patients, only approximately half of the patients revealed teratozoospermia. Surgery also did not induce a noticeable change in this situation. The morphology deteriorated in 12% of the patients, improved in an equal number, and remained unchanged in 64 patients (76%).

Carnitine Levels in Seminal Plasma (Table 4)

Carnitine values were determined in seminal plasma of 23 patients preceeding and following varicocele surgery. The carnitine level was reduced in 12 patients prior to surgery, and only 7 thereafter. This would indicate that the level of carnitine increases with increasing sperm density.

Discussion

The results of the present study are consistent with the majority of the existing publications with regard to sperm density [1–6, 10, 12–14, 17–19, review at 9]. Since a significant positive correlation between sperm density and carnitine level has frequently been observed [8, 21], normalization of the carnitine level in seminal plasma can also be expected postoperatively in cases with improved sperm density. This conclusion is also supported by our results.

With respect to motility, we have obtained less favorable postoperative results than most of the previous investigators [2, 7, 11–13, 15, 17, 19]. Our results correspond to those of only a few authors [3, 5].

In most cases, the sperm morphology in our varicocele patients was not influenced by surgery, similar to the reports of Haensch [7] and Mauss et al. [13]. The morphological alterations designated by MacLeod [11, 12], as varicocele-typical (tapering forms) were not revealed in such a manner in our patients.

A hydrocele can occur as a complication of varicocele surgery, as we observed in 6 of our 84 cases (7%). Wallijn and Desmet [20] reported an equal rate; the percentages of Charny [3] and Scott and Young [17] were lower.

The overall outcome of the present study is not satisfactory because it does not provide a clear indication of the actual value of surgical treatment of a varicocele. We feel that our results basically do not differ from those of the previously published studies. We have prepared this communication in order to point out the fundamental problems of such reports in a competent forum. The substantial deviation in results has already been referred to in the previous contribution (H. Kasseckert and W. Adam see this vol. p 41).

In our opinion, the postoperative results of ejaculate parameters will continue to be of limited significance as long as the manner in which ejaculate quality is impaired by varicoceles cannot be determined on the basis of concrete clinical findings on individual patients; in other words, until uniform criteria of evaluation [cf. 16] are established with which a follow-up study of a large group of patients can be performed by different investigators. And then, of course, it still will not be possible to exclude all interfering factors, the most important of which is the "part" of the female partner. Yet in this manner it would be possible to obtain a sufficiently large group of patients to permit decent statistical evaluation.

References

1. Brauss H, Klein P (1971) Über eine operative Behandlung der Varicocele. Grosse, Berlin (Fortschr Fert Forsch vol II) pp 139–141
2. Brown JS (1976) Varicocelectomy in the subfertile man: A ten-year experience with 295 cases. Fertil Steril 27:1046–1053
3. Charny CW (1962) Effect of varicocele on fertility. Results of varicocelectomy. Fertil Steril 13:47–56
4. Dubin L, Amelar RD (1975) Varicocelectomy as therapy in male infertility: A study of 504 cases. Fertil Steril 26:217–220
5. Gall H, Schnierstein H, Glowania H-J (1979) Fertilitätsverbesserung beim Mann durch Varikozelenoperation? Eine Studie an 100 subfertilen Varikozelepatienten 3 Monate nach der Operation. Urologe [A] 18:183–186
6. Glezerman M, Rakowszczyk M, Lunenfeld B, Beer R, Goldman B (1976) Varicocele in oligospermic patients: Pathophysiology and results after ligation and division of the internal spermatic vein. J Urol 115:562–565
7. Haensch R (1976) Der Einfluß der Varikozelenoperation nach Palomo auf das Spermiogramm. Hautarzt 27:449–452
8. Hook B, Adam W, Deichsel G (1981) Zum Aussagewert von Carnitin- und Citratbestimmung im Seminalplasma. In: Schirren C, Mettler L, Semm K (eds) Grosse, Berlin (Fortschr Fert Forsch 8) pp 159–161
9. Jecht E (1977) Varikozele und Fertilität. Übersichtsarbeit. Z Haut Geschlechtskr 138:177–187
10. Ludvik W (1970) Varikozele und Fertilität. Aktuel Urol 1:184–192
11. MacLeod J (1965) Seminal cytology in the presence of varicocele. Fertil Steril 16:735–757
12. MacLeod J (1969) Further observations in the role of varicocele in human male infertility. Fertil Steril 20:545–563
13. Mauss J, Schach H, Scheidt J (1974) Andrologische Untersuchungen bei subfertilen Männern vor und nach Varicocelenoperation. Hautarzt 25:394–398
14. Meyhöfer W, Wolf J (1960) Varikozele und Fertilität. Dermatol Wochenschr 142:1116–1121
15. Rost A, Richter-Reichhelm M, Kaden R, Pust R (1976) Effekt der operativen Varikozelentherapie auf die Spermiogenese. Grosse, Berlin (Fortschr Fert Forsch Bd III) pp 67–70
16. Schirren JM (1971) Methodenkritische Bemerkungen zu einer andrologischen Gemeinschaftsuntersuchung. Methods Inform Med 10:148–155
17. Scott LS, Young D (1962) Varicocele: a study of its effects on human spermatogenesis, and of the results produced by spermatic vein ligation. Fertil Steril 13:325–334
18. Tulloch WS (1955) Varicocele in subfertility: results of treatment. Br Med J II:356–358
19. Völter D, Knoth W, Lüders G (1971) Die Varikozelenoperation nach Giuliani. Dtsch Med Wochenschr 96:641–644
20. Wallijn E, Desmet R (1978) Hydrocele: A frequently overlooked complication after high ligation of the spermatic vein for varicocele. Int J Andrology 1:411–415
21. Wetterauer U, Heite H-J (1976) Der Carnitin-Gehalt im Sperma – ein Parameter für die Nebenhodenfunktion. Aktuel Dermatol 3:93–103

Treatment of Idiopathic Varicoceles by Transfemoral Testicular Vein Occlusion

L. Weissbach, M. Thelen, and H.-D. Adolphs

Introduction

A varicocele is operated on according to methods described by Ivanissevich, Bernardi, or Palomo. The failure rate is 0.2%–25% [2, 5, 8].

The venous drainage of the testis can be visualized by means of phlebography before surgical ligation of the testicular vein.

Only the transfemoral technique with probing of the renal vein permits reflux of contrast medium into the testicular vein, thus providing evidence of the pathological hemodynamics of the insufficient venous system. With additional selective probing of the testicular vein, possible collateral circulations are diagnosed. The high rate of recurrence or persistence after operations on the varicoceles have prompted us to perform embolization immediately after transfemoral phlebography.

Method

After puncture of the right femoral vein in the groin, the angiographic catheter is inserted via the inferior vena cava into the left renal vein. The venous reflux is shown and documented. The testicular vein is then probed far enough that the proximal end of the foreign body to be applied does not reach into the lumen of the renal vein. For occlusion, we use the Gianturco coil [3]. Thrombotic occlusion of the vessel occurs within 20 min.

Patients

We occluded the left testicular vein because of an idiopathic varicocele in a total of 22 patients. In 15 cases, we were able to conduct long-term follow-up studies over an average period of 11.5 months. In four of the follow-up studies, a total of six unsuccessful operations had been performed. To evaluate the long-term results, the following investigations were carried out: recording of the interim history, clinical status, plate thermography, i.v. urography, control phlebography, and spermiogram.

Results

Three patients were lost to follow-up. In four further cases, treatment results could only be evaluated within a period of 3 weeks to 3 months. At this time, the varicocele could no longer be palpated. In the remaining patients, we were able to perform long-term follow-up studies.

Interim History

Five patients displayed transient pain symptoms in the left flank or left groin. Two other patients complained of persistent pain which we attributed to a discrete ingui-

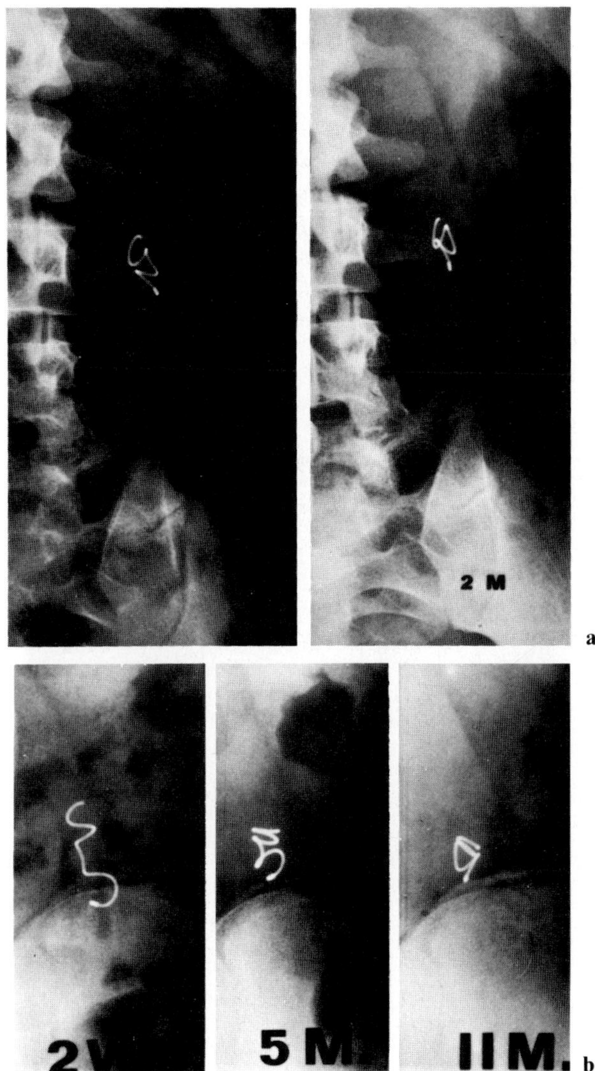

Fig. 1. a Change of configuration of the Gianturco coil during 2 months. *Left*: original situation after embolization, *right*: 2 months later. **b** Change of configuration after 5 and 11 months, respectively.

nal hernia. A 31-year-old patient suffered from pain symptoms more than 12 months after embolization. The foreign body applied was removed by partial resection of the testicular vein. Today, this patient still reports diffuse pain in the lower abdomen; he is receiving psychiatric treatment.

Clinical Findings

Thirteen of fifteen patients show a complete remission of the previously ectatic pampiniform plexus. In two boys, the varicocele was still (n = 1) and again (n = 1) demonstrable 1 year after embolization.

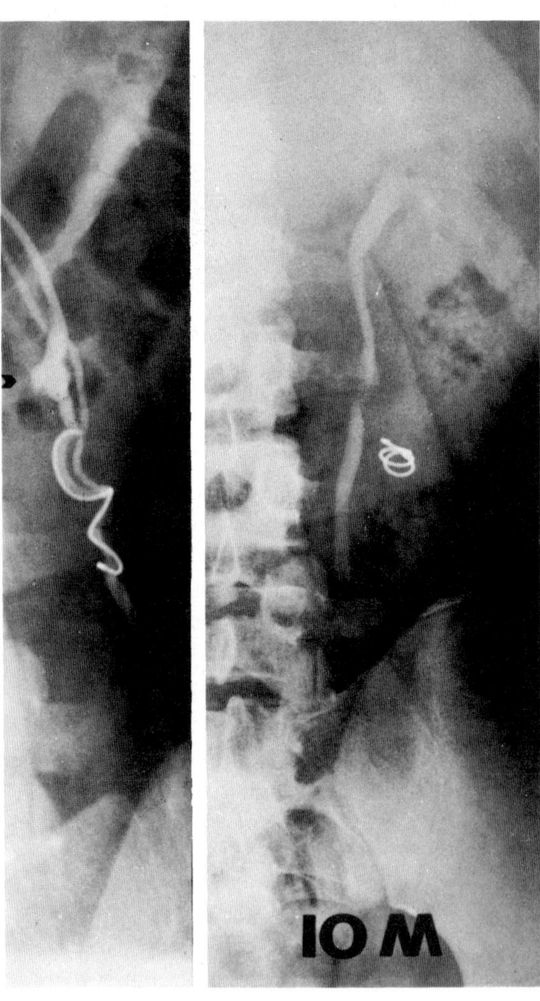

Fig. 2. *Left*: Application of Gianturco coil in one branch of the testicular vein with craniocaudal flow of the opacified blood; venous branch parallel to this vessel with sufficient valve (*arrow*). *Right*: Position of the metal coil lateral to the ureter.

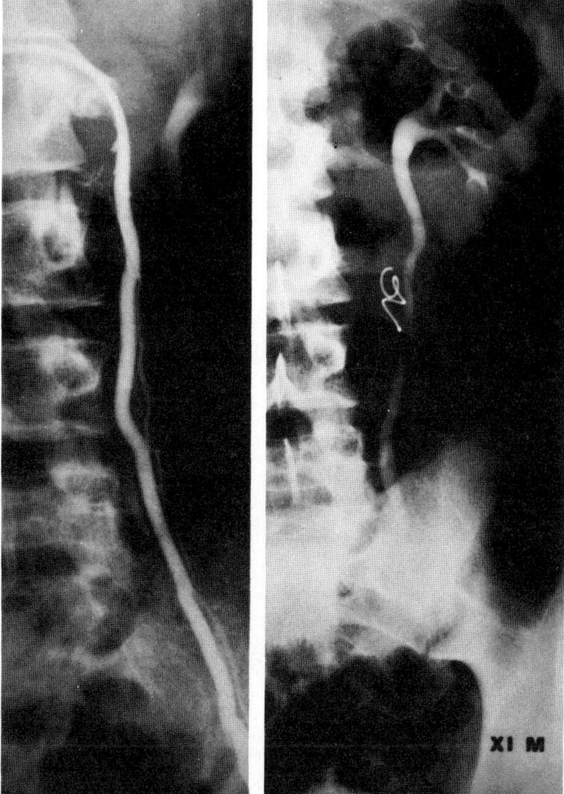

Fig. 3. *Left*: Transfemoral phlebography in idiopathic varicocele with follow-up intravenous urography 11 months later. *Right*: Position of the metal coil medial to the ureter.

Plate Thermography

In the two unsuccessfully treated cases, the temperature was still markedly raised over the left scrotum. The patient with persistent inguinal pain still had a slightly elevated temperature, although the varicocele had already regressed. In all other cases, there was no temperature difference between the two sides of the scrotum.

Radiologic Findings

Radiographic controls were performed in all 15 patients 1 year after embolization. Almost all coils changed in length compared with the original measurements. A distinct shortening already occurred within 8 weeks and became even more pronounced during the course of a year (Fig. 1). The coil projects at the site of the original application; no dislocation occurs.

In i.v. urography, the coil is found lateral to the ureter in most cases (Fig. 2). The metal body is only rarely located medial to the ureter (Fig. 3). In a patient with a

    L. Weißbach et al.

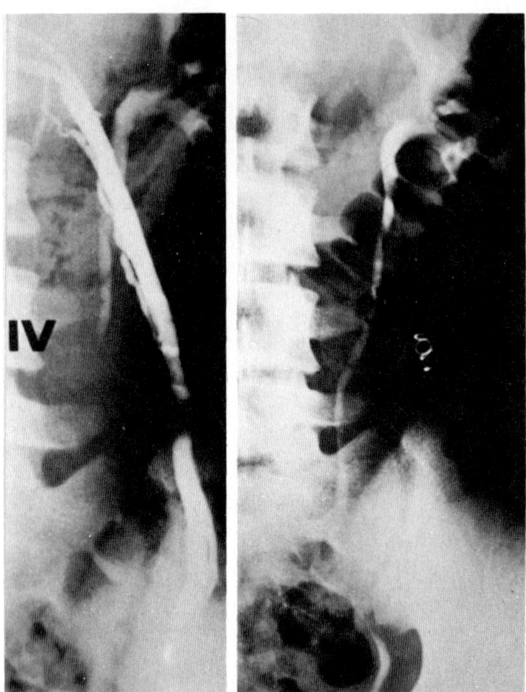

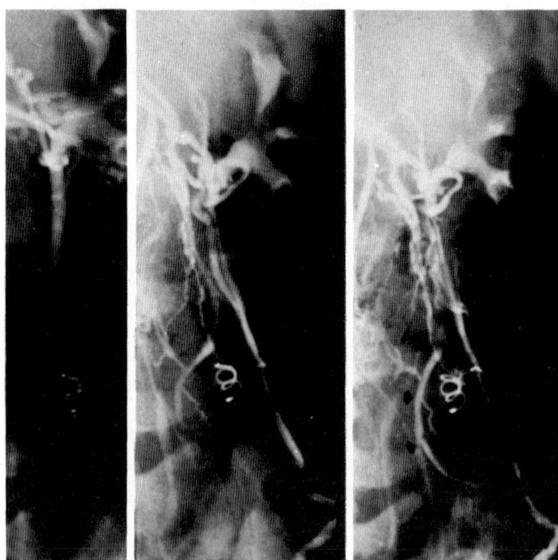

Fig. 4. a *Left*: Original phlebogram in a patient with varicocele. Suspicion of a tiny collateral vein at the level of the IVth vertebral body. *Right*: Control urography 1 year later. **b** Extensive development of collateral veins 1 year after embolization. (arrows)

recurrent varicocele after embolization, we were able to perform a control phlebography, thus demonstrating the development of a collateral circulation (Fig. 4).

Spermiogram

In nine patients, an examination of the ejaculate had to be dispensed with because of the lack of sexual maturity. Two patients with oligozoospermia reported conceptions 4–6 months later. Two patients showed a normozoospermia and four an oligozoospermia.

Discussion

Embolization or sclerotization can be performed as an alternative to surgical treatment of varicocele. Advantages of these percutaneous treatment techniques are: no requirement for general anesthesia, a specific occlusion of the insufficient veins after phlebography, and shortening of the hospital stay. If a sclerosing agent is injected via a catheter into the testicular vein, simultaneous occlusion of further anastomosing veins is advantageous [4, 9]. The local finding in the scrotum occasionally indicated a reflux of the slcerosing agent into the pampiniform plexus [6, 9]. The embolization is performed with the metal coil [7] or detachable balloons [1]. In multiple veins, each vessel can be occluded separately; in anastomosis , a pinpointed occlusion can be effected at the confluence. The embolization material must meet important requirements for application in a vein: no dislocation, lasting occlusion, no foreign body reaction, radiological detectability.

References

1. Barth KH, White RI Jr (1980) Occlusion with detachable balloons. This volume page 152
2. Dubin L, Amelar RD (1975) Varicocelectomy as therapy in male infertility: A study of 504 cases. Fertil Steril 26:217
3. Gianturco C, Anderson JH, Wallace S (1975) Mechanical devices for arterial occlusion. Am J Roentgenol 124:428
4. Iaccarino V (1977) Trattamento conservativo del varicocele: Flebografie selettiva e sclero- terapia delle vene gonadiche. Riv Radiol 17:107
5. Lindholmer C, Thulin L, Eliasson R (1975) Semen characteristica before and after ligation of the left internal spermatic veins in men with varicocele. Scand J Urol Nephrol 9:177
6. Riedl P (1979) Selektive Phlebographie und Katheterthrombosierung der Vena testicularis bei primärer Varikozele. Wien Klin Wochenschr 91:3
7. Thelen M, Weißbach L, Franken Th (1979) Die Behandlung der idiopathischen Varikozele durch transfemorale Spiralokklusion der Vena testicularis sinistra. ROEFO 131:24
8. Weißbach L (1978) Die idiopathische Varikozele – Eine Übersicht. Extract Urol 1:255
9. Zeitler E, Jecht E, Richter E-I, Seyferth W (1980) Perkutane Behandlung männlicher In- fertilität im Rahmen der selektiven Spermatikaphlebographie. ROEFO 132:294

Effect of Percutaneous Sclerosis of the Left Internal Spermatic Vein on Semen Quality

E. W. Jecht, E.-I. Richter, W. Seyferth, and E. Zeitler

There is general agreement that reduced semen quality will improve following varicocele operation – "high ligation" – in more than 50% of patients with a varicocele [3, 9]. Lima et al. [5] have demonstrated that selective sclerosis will interrupt a retrograde flow in the internal spermatic vein. We previously used selective phlebography of the internal spermatic vein as a diagnostic technique [10, see also this symposium]. Since sclerosis can be accomplished "without any significant prolongation of the diagnostic procedure" [5], we decided to occlude the internal spermatic vein where necessary and feasible.

Percutaneous selective sclerosis of the left internal spermatic vein was performed in 69 patients with evidence of retrograde flow in this blood vessel. The technique of this intervention has been reported previously [11]. We here present a preliminary analysis of the pre- and postocclusive seminal parameters in these 69 patients. A conclusive evaluation of the effect of sclerosis on semen quality must await larger numbers of patients so treated.

Table 1. Semen quality prior to and following sclerosis of the left internal spermatic vein ($n = 69$)

Variable	$\bar{x}_1$ Preocclusive	$\bar{x}_2$ Postocclusive	n
Count ($\times 10^6$/ml)	26.34	31.51 [a]	63
Motility (% motile)	47.85	49.65	65
Morphology (% normal)	40.74	43.26 [a]	65

[a] $P < 0.05$

Table 2. Semen quality prior to and following sclerosis of the left internal spermatic vein ($n = 12$)

Variable	$\bar{x}_1$ Preocclusive	$\bar{x}_2$ Postocclusive	n
Count ($\times 10^6$/ml)	11.2	24.2 [a]	12
Motility (% motile)	46	54 [a]	12
Morphology (% normal)	41.3	43.3	12

[a] $P < 0.01$

Table 3. Semen quality prior to and following sclerosis of the left internal spermatic vein ($n=43$)

Variable	$\bar{x}_1$ Preocclusive	$\bar{x}_2$ Postocclusive	n
Count ($\times 10^6$/ml)	23.74	30.31 [a]	43
Motility (% motile)	43.7	49.5 [a]	40
Morphology (% normal)	39.84	43.24	39

[a] $P < 0.001$

Table 4. Degenerative cells and spermatogenic cells prior to and following sclerosis of the left internal spermatic vein ($n=69$)

Variable	$\bar{x}_1$ Preocclusive	$\bar{x}_2$ Postocclusive	n
Spermatogenic cells (%)	4.44	2.75 [a]	62
Degenerative cells (%)	25.6	14.6 [b]	64

[a] $P < 0.05$
[b] $P < 0.005$

The mean values of sperm count, motility, and morphology both before and following sclerosis are summarized in Table 1. There is a definite tendency towards improvement of all three seminal variables; for two variables (count and morphology) a (relatively weak) statistical significance can be shown ($P = 0.05$, Wilcoxon matched-pairs signed-ranks test [8]).

It is worth repeating that the data in Table 1 are based on too small a number of patients. As demonstrated by the data obtained for the first 12 (Table 2) and 43 (Table 3) patients treated by sclerosis, the high intraindividual variation of seminal parameters [7] can easily lead to deceptive results. The postocclusive improvement appears much more pronounced for the two smaller groups ($P \leqq 0.01$ for count and motility) than for the 69 patients (Table 1). The lapse of time from sclerosis to postocclusive semen analysis plays, of course, an important role not sufficiently taken into account by this presentation.

In 1978, we introduced the degenerative cells as a seminal variable characteristic for the presence of a varicocele [4]. We were, therefore, particularly interested in studying the influence of sclerosis on these cells as well as on the spermatogenic cells [6]. The highly significant ($P \leqq 0.005$) postocclusive reduction of degenerative cells (Table 4) appears to confirm our assumption regarding the relation of these seminal elements to varicocele. Spermatogenic cells also showed a significant ($P \geqq 0.05$) postocclusive decrease; their incidence, however, was already relatively small before sclerosis.

Most investigators have reported an improvement of semen quality in 60% [1] to 70% [2] following high ligation. Our data do not bear out such a high rate of improvement, the percentages being 40% (count/ml, motility, morphology) and 50% (total sperm count). Whether this difference is due to the relatively small number of patients studied (cf. 1: 251 patients, 2: 504 patients) and/or the short time interval from occlusion to postocclusive semen analysis (3 months for 29 patients) remains to be seen.

The unequivocal postocclusive reduction of degenerative cells is, to us, a clear demonstration for the efficacy of sclerosis in treating varicoceles. Therefore, we expect a further improvement of our results as more patients are included at longer time intervals after occlusion. In conclusion, we feel that percutaneous selective sclerosis is as efficient as high ligation and at the same time much simpler since performed as an outpatient procedure [11].

References

1. Brown JS (1976) Varicocelectomy in the subfertile male: A ten-year experience with 295 cases. Fertil Steril 27:1046
2. Dubin L, Amelar RD (1975) Varicocelectomy as therapy in male infertility: study of 504 cases. Fertil Steril 26:217
3. Jecht E (1977) Varikozele und Fertilität. Z Haut Geschlechtskr 138:177
4. Jecht E (1978) Indikationen zur hohen Ligatur der Vena spermatica interna aus der Sicht des dermatologischen Andrologen. Therapiewoche 28:1905
5. Lima SS, Castro MP, Costa OF (1978) A new method for the treatment of varicocele. Andrologia 10:103
6. MacLeod J (1965) Seminal cytology in the presence of varicocele. Fertil Steril 16:735
7. Schwartz D, Laplanche A, Jouannet P, David G (1979) Within-subject variability of human semen in regard to sperm count, volume, total number of spermatozoa and length of abstinence. J Reprod Fertil 57:391
8. Siegel S (1956) Nonparametric statistics for the behavioral sciences. McGraw Hill, New York Toronto London
9. Verstoppen GR, Steeno OP (1977) Varicocele and the pathogenesis of the associated subfertility. A review of the various theories. II. Results of surgery. Andrologia 9:293
10. Zeitler E, Jecht E, Herzinger R, Richter E-I, Seyferth W, Grosse-Vorholt R (1979) Technik und Ergebnisse der Spermatica-Phlebographie bei 136 Männern mit primärer Sterilität. ROEFO 131:179
11. Zeitler E, Jecht E, Richter E-I, Seyferth W (1980) Perkutane Behandlung männlicher Infertilität im Rahmen der selektiven Spermatikaphlebographie mit Katheter. ROEFO 132:294

VII. Discussion

Phlebography of Persistent Varicocele in Boys

T. Riebel

Few cases of scrotal varicocele are known in pediatrics. Øster [3] first reported varicoceles in the age group of 10 years and above when examining 1072 healthy Danish schoolboys. Various other references confirm his findings of the average incidence of 16% in 10–19 year old boys (Table 1). Janneck [2], in his paper on 43 children with idiopathic varicocele, reports on 12 boys who developed a varicocele as early as between 4 and 9 years of age.

After high ligation of the testicular vein, 1%–3% of cases show no improvement of the varicose dilatation of the veins around the testicle. In order to obtain information on nonligated trunks of the spermatic vein as well as indications of hemodynamically important collaterals, our urologists and pediatric surgeons prefer phlebography for boys with persistent varicocele. Access and operative procedure can be planned more exactly and, consequently, the children can be better protected from further fertility impairment.

Based on a series of roentgenograms taken during the examinations of children, the technique and results of the retrograde spermatica-phlebography will be shown; this technique is neither very burdening nor very complicated for this group of patients.

Patient I. 11-year-old boy with postoperative continuous painful dilatation of the veins around the left testicle. After the percutaneous puncture of the right femoral vein performed according to Seldinger, a catheter is pushed forward through the external and common iliac veins and the inferior vena cava into the left renal vein, and further to the orifice area of the left internal spermatic vein. Then,

Table 1. Incidence of varicocele

Author	Examined healthy men		% Cases with varicocele
	Number	Age (years)	
Oster (3)	1072	6 – 19	16.2
	188	6 – 19	0
	53	10	5.7
	207	14	19.3
Horner (1)		15	20.5
Steeno et al. (4)	4076	12 – 15	14.7
German army recruitment	3 million		17.0

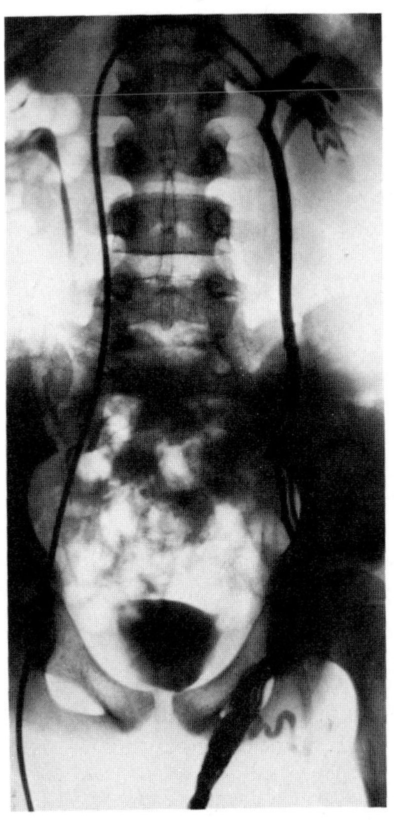

Fig. 1. 11-year-old boy with left-sided varicocele. Spermatica-phlebography of persistence before reoperation.

with the patient in a more upright position, the contrast medium is injected. This can reach the pampiniform plexus only in the case of varicocele, as a result of the reversal of blood circulation through the testicular vein. In addition to the normal intrarenal veins, a strong, valveless vascular trunk which was left open during the operation, is shown with a short-distanced filling of the cranial portion of the ligated spermatic vein branch (Fig. 1). Distal are 2, in the inguinal channel 4 and more varicose trunks of the testicular vein present. The pampiniform plexus is clearly dilated because of the persistent varicocele. We see strong collateral flowing-off of the contrast medium through the external pudendal vein to the left femoral vein and on to the iliac vein. Reoperation with ligation of the angiographically shown open spermatic vein branches leads to positive result.

Patient II. 13-year-old boy with persistent left-sided varicocele. Percutaneous catheterization of the testicular vein via the right femoral and pelvic vein, the inferior vena cava, and the left renal vein was performed. After the patient had been brought to an upright position, the contrast medium was injected. In addition to inconspicuous filling of intrarenal veins and the renal vein, the rich flow of the contrast medium extended to the scrotum through a spermatic vein trunk (Fig. 2a). In the middle vascular segment, a short joining vessel can be demonstrated, which rep-

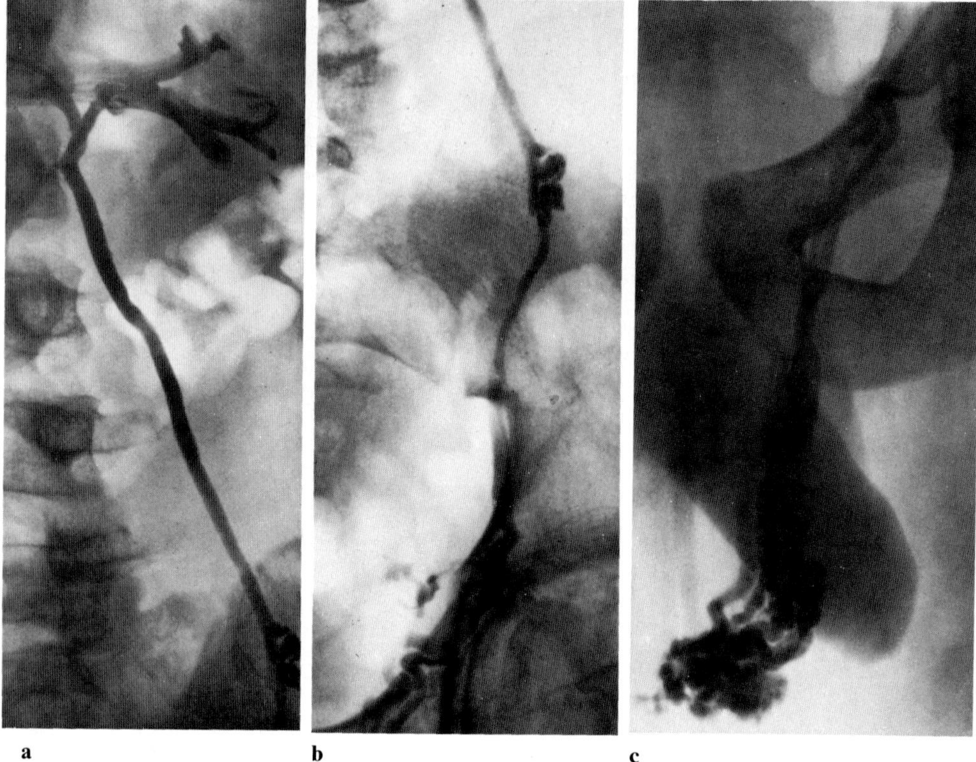

a   b   c

Fig. 2 a–c. 13-year-old boy with persistent left-sided varicocele. Phlebographic demonstration.

resents the cranial portion of the testicular vein segment ligated earlier. Distal to it, collaterals to pelvic veins are slightly contrasted (Fig. 2 b). Two strong vascular trunks are seen in the inguinal channel. The pampiniform plexus is dilated and grossly tortuous. No further collaterals are seen (Fig. 2 c). When reoperating upon the patient later, ligation of the two testicular vein trunks still open was performed.

Patient III. 11-year-old boy. As with the other two patients, an intravenous urogram showed no cause for a secondary varicocele. The technique of the left-sided spermatica phlebography was similar to that used on the other two patients. The orifice area of the vein was free. Retrograde injection of contrast medium revealed a valveless strong and another thinner trunk of the spermatic vein. Partial filling of the ureteric vein occurred. In the inguinal channel were several vascular trunks of the testicular vein present. The pampiniform plexus appeared varicosely changed. Altogether, no collateral circulation was noticed. A second operation produced positive results.

Method, indication, and value of the phlebographic demonstration of persistent varicocele as well as the venous flowing-off condition were to be explained by these case reviews. The advantage of examination for the necessary reoperation in children should be emphasized.

References

1. Horner JS (1960) The varicocele. A survey amongst secondary school boys. Medical Officer 104:377
2. Janneck C (1979) Varikozele im Kindesalter. Chir Praxis 25:323
3. Øster J (1971) Varicocele in children and adolescents. Scand J Urol Nephrol 5:27
4. Steeno O, Knops J, Declerck L, Adimoelja A, van de Voorde H (1976) Prevention of fertility disorders by detection and treatment of varicocele at school age. Andrologia 8:52

Subject Index

T. Mann, C. Lutwak-Mann

Male Reproductive Function and Semen

Themes and Trends in Physiology, Biochemistry and Investigate Andrology

1981. 46 figures. XIV, 495 pages
ISBN 3-540-10383-X

Contents: Male Reproductive Function and the Composition of Semen: General Considerations. – Methodological Guidelines in the Study of Male Reproductive Organs. – Collection, Examination, Quality Rating and Storage of Ejaculated Semen. – Testis and Testicular Semen. – Epididymis and Epididymal Semen. – Vas Deferens and Vasectomy. – Secretory Function of the Prostate, Seminal Vesicle, Cowper's Gland and Other Accessory Organs of Reproduction. – Biochemistry of Spermatozoa: Chemical and Functional Correlations in Ejaculated Semen, Andrological Aspects. – Biochemistry of Seminal Plasma and Male Accessory Fluids; Application to Andrological Problems. – Effects of Pharmacological Agents: Andrological Aspects. Drug Abuse, Therapeutic Agents, Male Contraceptives, Occupational Hazards. – References. – Subject Index.

The prodigious expansion in the physiological and biochemistry of male reproduction function since the appearance of Biochemistry of Semen and of the Male Reproductive Tract in 1964 makes a coherent and meaningful survey of research endeavour in this area extremely timely. Themselves responsible for much of this expansion, Drs. Mann and Mann have drawn upon their own vast experience to provide the scientific community with just such a critical overview. They highlight new investigative techniques and selected topics which show how advances in this field are contributing to the development of clinical and investigative andrology in both human and veterinary medicine. The comparative approach is adopted in describing normal reproductive processes, illustrated by examples drawn from studies on both man and animals. Abnormal aspects are also covered, among them spermatogenic failure, hormonal disarray, malfunction of male accessory glands, and pathological changes in sperm plasmalemma, acrosome, nucleus, mitochondria, flagellum, and the seminal plasma. Special attention is given to adverse effects of pharmacological agents upon both human and animal reproductive function and semen. This book will prove an invaluable source of information not only for researchers engaged in the study of mammalian and non-mammalian reproduction, but also for clinical and research urologists and andrologists, veterinarians, and teachers and advanced students of the physiology of reproduction.

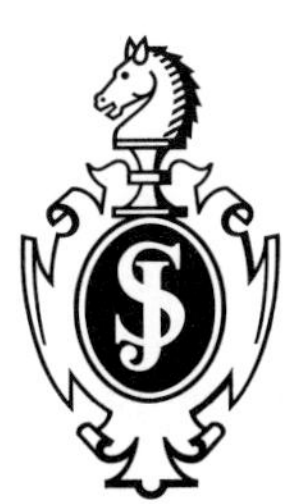

Springer-Verlag
Berlin
Heidelberg
New York